The Meaning of the
Dream in Psychoanalysis

SUNY series in Dream Studies
Robert L. Van de Castle, editor

THE MEANING
OF THE DREAM
IN PSYCHOANALYSIS

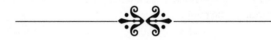

Rachel B. Blass

STATE UNIVERSITY OF NEW YORK PRESS

Published by
State University of New York Press, Albany

© 2002 State University of New York

For information, address State University of New York Press,
90 State Street, Suite 700, Albany, NY, 12207

Production by Marilyn P. Semerad
Marketing by Patrick Durocher

Library of Congress Cataloging-in-Publication Data

Blass, Rachel B., 1961–
    The meaning of the dream in psychoanalysis / Rachel B. Blass.
        p. cm. — (SUNY series in dream studies)
    Includes bibliographical references and index
    ISBN 0–7914–5317–0 (alk. paper)—ISBN 0–7914–5318–9 (pbk. : alk. paper)
    1. Dream interpretation. 2. Dreams. 3. Psychoanalysis. I. Title. II. Series.

BF175.5D74 B57 2002
154.6′3—dc21
                                                                    2001042012

10 9 8 7 6 5 4 3 2 1

CONTENTS

ACKNOWLEDGMENTS

This book was made possible in part by grants from the Israel Foundation Trustees. Chapter 2 incorporates some ideas I expressed in my paper "The Limitations of Critical Studies of the Epistemology of Freud's Dream Theory and their Clinical Implications," which appears in *Psychoanalysis and Contemporary Thought,* 24 (2001). I am thankful to International Universities Press for permission to use that material.

Introduction

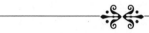

> Books are the entryway to dreams.
> —Fernando Pessoa, *The Book of Disquiet*

From the time of antiquity the dream has mystified humankind. The desire to know the meaning of the images that pass through our mind in the course of sleep, the meaning of the strange events that happen to us then, and the stories with which we wake up and have been waking up since childhood, have led over the generations to a range of theories regarding the dream and its meaning. Many of these theories may be read as warnings to those who wish to penetrate the mystery: "There is nothing to be sought there, the dream has no meaning." Freud (1856–1939), more than any other modern-day investigator, would not heed such warnings. He took it upon himself to discover the meaning of the apparently meaningless; to reveal the secrets of the mind that seem to elude comprehension. It was his ardent wish to know the dream, for him a last bastion of mental products that seemed to refuse to succumb to human understanding.

Freud asserts that it was on July 24, 1895, that "the secret of the dream revealed itself to Dr. Sigm. Freud" (Freud, 1985, p. 417). It was approximately five years later that he published his most comprehensive statement on this revelation, appearing in his best-known book *The Interpretation of Dreams* (1900). There he presents in detail what were to become the foundations and the heart of the psychoanalytic theory regarding the meaning of dreams.

The present book comes to critically examine this theory. The question it deals with is an epistemological one: What is the justification for the assertion that we know or can come to know a meaning of a dream? To further demar-

1

cate: The question is not whether the dream has this or that particular meaning, but rather whether it is possible to obtain any knowledge regarding the meaning of the dream. That is, the question is *whether there is any support at all to the idea that dream analysis can lead to the discovery of meanings that actually exist in the dream.* If the dream does have meaning, can we indeed come to know of it, as Freud and all of his followers to the present day so strongly affirm?

Although I am here putting into question a major tenet of psychoanalytic thought, this is not my aim per se. This study is not another in the series of works aimed at uprooting or demolishing Freudian psychoanalysis piece by piece (e.g., Eysenck, 1985; Eysenck & Wilson, 1973; Masson, 1984). On the contrary, in the course of the study I will take as a basic premise that the psychoanalytic theory as a whole is valid and justified. Although this premise may seem far-reaching, it allows me to examine epistemological issues specific to the dream theory that arise from within the psychoanalytic framework. As I will show, assuming the general validity of this framework, there emerge special obstacles to the justification of the psychoanalytic dream theory that have been neglected in the psychoanalytic and philosophical literature. Both the study of the difficulties that this specific theory faces and the way in which I believe they may be overcome, at least in part, may be seen to have not only theoretical significance, but clinical significance as well.

This book will be composed of six chapters. In chapter 1, I will prepare the ground for various issues dealt with throughout the book. This preparation first entails the clarification of some basic terms, primarily the terms of justification and meaning. We must have some conception regarding what constitutes a justification if we are to inquire into the justification of the psychoanalytic theory regarding the meaning of the dream. We must also have some conception of the meaning of meaning. Both terms are complex, involving matters of definition as well as views regarding epistemology and what psychoanalysis is all about.

The emergence of a hermeneuticist approach within psychoanalysis in the past twenty-five years has led to some confusion regarding the range of available forms of justification as well as regarding the meaning of meaning. The psychoanalytical hermeneuticists argue that the scientific approach is not relevant to psychoanalysis, which is concerned with meaning, and that the limited empirical methods of justification, which are applicable to the natural sciences have no place when it comes to this unique theory of meaning. Most importantly, in their view, the meanings of what we do, say, think, or express in some other way, are not the kinds of things that can be *discovered*; we cannot reveal the actual or true meanings that exist in the subject's mind. Rather, we attribute meanings to our expressions either on the basis of some *creative* literary analysis of them or on the basis of our *descriptions* of our immediate experience of what these meanings are. But there is no inherent connection between these creative and descriptive attributions of meaning and anything that really exists within us and can be discovered. Thus to adopt these views of justification and meaning is to dismiss the very framework within which there emerges our epistemological question regarding the possibility of discovering the meanings of dreams.

It is for this reason that in clarifying the terms "justification" and "meaning" I have found it necessary to discuss this hermeneuticist approach, as well as the hermeneuticists' view of the scientific approach that they consider themselves to be contending with, an approach often referred to as "positivistic." By clarifying the hermeneuticist claims against "positivism" I will sharpen the conceptualizations of these terms in psychoanalysis today. This will also bring to the fore how—contrary to the hermeneuticist position—psychoanalysis as a theory of meaning may remain within the sphere of science and apply various suitable forms of justification. It is thus possible and important to inquire into the question of whether we are discovering the true meanings of our expressions, including the true meanings of our dreams.

Having clarified these terms, I will turn to a brief overview of Freud's uses of the term "meaning" and "justification" as well as to the related term "truth."

Finally, I will examine the works of two writers who have specifically raised epistemological questions regarding the psychoanalytic theory of dream interpretation (Grünbaum, 1984, 1993; Spence, 1981). This will point to the place and necessity of the current study.

Chapter 2 turns to Freud and the foundations that he set for the psychoanalytic theory of dream interpretation. The bulk of the chapter is a careful and comprehensive critical analysis of Freud's argument in favor of the dream theory as he set it forth in his *The Interpretation of Dreams* (1900). I will show how his justification of the theory does not stand up to the criteria that Freud himself set. But I will also show how this failure does not necessitate the rejection of the dream theory or a hermeneutical modification of it such that it may be accepted even though it does not really tell us anything regarding meanings that actually exist in the dream. I will argue, rather, that this failure points to another possible source of justification. Although Freud did not present or fully recognize it as such, the justification of the dream theory ultimately relies on its belonging to the broader network of psychoanalytic thinking. While it cannot stand on its own right, it may derive its validity from its place in the broader network of ideas. The dream theory is in effect an application of general psychoanalytic thought and method to the dream, rather than an independent theory with its own methods.

The fact that dream interpretation involves the application of general psychoanalytic principles to the dream may not come as news to any practitioner. However, the recognition of the fact that the *justification* of the theory rests solely on this application does raise a crucial issue that has not been addressed:

Is the application of general psychoanalytic principles to the dream legitimate? This cannot be taken for granted.

Chapter 3 sets forth the basic principles and assumptions that underlie psychoanalysis' general theory of meaning. It then carefully examines whether it is legitimate to apply these principles and assumptions to the dream. Does the available evidence regarding the state of our psyche and its meanings during the dream warrant such an application? The conclusion is that basic phenomenological and commonsense observation put this in doubt. Relying on familiar evidence, the dream appears to hold a special status as a potential context of meaning that results from the unique difficulty in determining the nature of the network of meaning that is operative during the dream. If it cannot be determined that the same basic networks of meaning are operative during the dream and during the wakeful state in which the dream is being interpreted, then the general psychoanalytic principles for discovery of meaning cannot be applied to the dream.

If this conclusion is not overturned, then we will not have succeeded in putting forth a justification of the psychoanalytic theory of dreams. In the absence of the possibility of applying to the dream the general psychoanalytic principles for the discovery of meaning, the epistemology of the dream theory remains unfounded. It would then be necessary to maintain an agnostic stance regarding dream interpretation. Namely, we would have to maintain that it may be that the dream is meaningful, but that in applying the psychoanalytic method of interpretation to the dream we do not in fact know whether we are discovering meanings or simply inventing them.

At the end of chapter 3, I will suggest that by relying on a new kind of evidence there is a way of coming to know that the network of meaning that is present during the dream is, indeed, the same as that which exists in the wakeful state. Consequently, general psychoanalytic principles can be applied to the dream and the theory can be justified. But before turning to the detailed exposition of *my* solution to the epistemological problem that faces the psychoanalytic theory of dreams, it is necessary to address the question of whether since 1900 there have been any new developments within psychoanalytic theory regarding the dream that have made obsolete the need for a solution. Has the psychoanalytic theory of dreams changed in a fundamental way such that the difficulties in relation to Freud's theory are overcome or are no longer relevant? Has a new form of justification been put forth? This is the topic of chapter 4. Here I do not go in detail into the new approach to dream analysis that is put forth by psychoanalytical hermeneuticists—since it is merely a derivative of their general position regarding the discovery of meaning and justification that was addressed in chapter 1—but rather I focus on the other developments that have taken place in the field.

Indeed, there have been many kinds of specific developments regarding dreams, and it is recognized that the dream no longer holds the royal place that it did at the time of Freud. Nevertheless, in terms of the approach to meaning and justification, the developments and examinations have not been that numerous. The clinical and theoretical innovations that have been put forth have not modified the basic conceptions of the nature of meaning and the methods of its discovery in such a way that the Freudian conceptions of these are no longer relevant. And the changes that have been introduced all rely on the assumption that the dream is a context of meaning and that its meanings may be discovered by the awake individual. Little, however, has been done to justify this proposition. In fact, the only analyst to continue to pursue its justification after 1900 was Freud himself. And while he seems, at points, to have taken some important steps toward understanding the difficulties involved in the justification process, ultimately, Freud's later attempts do not secure a more firm foundation for his dream theory than does his failed 1900 justification. The task of justifying the psychoanalytic dream theory still remains with us.

In the next chapter I intend to meet this task. But before doing so I turn to examine at greater length one particular development that has emerged regarding the dream theory. This is the development of what I refer to as the Affective-Experiential approach to the meaning of the dream, an approach that places special emphasis on experiencing the dream, rather than on recognizing the ideational connections that underlie it. This approach does not in any way provide a solution to the problem of the justification of the psychoanalytic claim that the analysis of dreams can lead to the discovery of their meaning. Nevertheless, it is important to understand it in order to distinguish the experiential dimensions to which it refers from those that I will discuss in my solution to the problem.

I set forth this solution in chapter 5. It is based on the in-depth analysis of an experiential dimension that has never been discussed in the relevant literature. I have called this dimension the "experiential quality of meaningfulness." The understanding of the nature of this experience and what it tells us regarding the state of the psyche ultimately points to the fact that this experience could not be felt in relation to dreams were it not for the fact that the individual's network of meaning when awake and during the dream are the same. Since we do at times experience meaningfulness in relation to our dreams, we must conclude that these networks are indeed basically the same (although they seem to find different forms of manifest expression). This conclusion provides the basis for the application to the dream of the general psychoanalytic principles for the determination of meaning. Once the application of these principles to the dream is found to be legitimate, justification of the dream theory is attained.

In this form of justification what is shown is that the epistemological basis for the psychoanalytic theory of dreams is indeed as well founded as the psychoanalytic theory in general is. For skeptics regarding psychoanalysis this may not be saying much, but for all those who contend that the basis of psychoanalysis is grounded as well as for those who have a strong intuition that its basis one day will be grounded, this should come as cheering news.

The final chapter, chapter 6, will end with a discussion of implications. They extend far beyond a simple conclusion that Freud's theory has now been proven right. There is a range of clinical and theoretical implications as well as implications for the inherent tie between the clinical and theoretical domains. While it is commonly recognized that theory shapes the clinical practice, it is not as well recognized that philosophically oriented, meta-theoretical issues have a direct effect on it. I hope to show in the course of this book not only that they do have this effect but also that these issues can be dealt with in a way that lends psychoanalysis scientific respectability. We need not rely on intuition alone or create new nonscientific domains in order to make sense of what psychoanalysis does.

⁙

Before turning to the examination of the issues at hand, I would like to add two comments on the nature of this study. The first has to do with the nature of its basic framework. My basic framework is psychoanalytical. I am assuming the general truth of psychoanalytic theory and examining whether within that framework the dream theory is justified. To examine this I must of course be able to stand outside the theory and observe it critically. But this does not require that I respond to critiques of the dream theory that are based on skepticism regarding the very foundations of psychoanalysis in general, or to critiques that psychoanalysis has already addressed. In this context recent objections to the psychoanalytic theory of dreams that have come from circles of biological research are not in the scope of the present study. Since, however, Hobson's & McCarley's (Hobson, 1988; Hobson & McCarley, 1977; McCarley and Hobson, 1977) work in this area has made these objections particularly popular I will now briefly explain why their biological findings do not refute the psychoanalytic dream theory.

In a nutshell, Hobson's and McCarley offer a physiological account of how the dream, with all its peculiarities, comes into being. They claim that the dream is generated without the involvement of the forebrain area and hence does not involve consciousness. They thus conclude, in contradiction to Freud's psychological theory of dream formation, that ideas cannot be the driving force of dreams (Hobson & McCarley, 1977).

There have been numerous responses to this critique (Fischer, 1978; Foulkes, 1985; Grünbaum, 1984; Labruzza, 1978), but that of the sleep physiologist Vogel (1978) is the most comprehensive. Not only does he point to additional evidence indicating that indeed the forebrain is involved, but he also addresses the methodological problem with refuting such a psychological theory on biological grounds. To do so, it must be shown that the activated state of the areas of the brain that have been found to generate the dream are in no way correlated with the psychological states that are hypothesized to be responsible for the dream. Vogel argues that Hobson and McCarley have failed to show this.

Moreover, it should be noted that at the heart of Hobson's and McCarley's critique of Freudian theory lies the claim that the dream instigators are not ideas or wishes. This, however, does not interfere with the possibility that at a later point in the dreaming process the lower-level brain activation, which according to Hobson and McCarley does instigate the dream, will be modified by higher level brain activity. The consequence of this would be that while the dream is not *instigated* by ideas, it does, nevertheless, *express* ideas. In fact, in one lecture, Hobson admitted that due to such later activity it is definitely possible that the dream would be an expression of "Freudian meanings" (Hobson, 1991). Since our concern is with meanings that the dream contains or expresses, the biological critique of the psychoanalytic dream theory, which centers on the issue of the original instigation of the dream, is irrelevant here. In fact, I would argue that it is irrelevant in general. As we will see, the essence of the psychoanalytic theory of dreams is in the claim that the dream contains accessible meanings. The claim that the nature of those meanings is wishes is secondary, and the claim that wishes are what *instigated* the dream is even further removed. (In 1933, even Freud [1993a, p. 29] directly puts forth the view that the wishful nature of dreams emerges from the processing of memory traces that arise in the dream simply because they are highly charged.)

I believe that the recent concern with the biological critiques of Freudian dream theory diverts attention from much more serious questions that currently threaten its foundations. The present study will bring these to the fore.

The second comment that I would like to make before turning to the study itself is about its form. In order to carefully analyze the nature of the dream theory and other related psychoanalytic formulations, such as various psychoanalytic formulations of meaning, truth, the process of interpretation, and so on, I have found it necessary to dissect broad psychoanalytic statements and propositions into very small parts. The clinical reader, who is not familiar with complex philosophical argumentation and who is acquainted with these psychoanalytic statements and propositions only in their broad form, may at first find it difficult to recognize them when viewed "under the microscope." An immediate reaction may be that this is "not what we are doing in our psychoanalytic work" or "this is not what we are saying through the psychoanalytic positions we have adopted." For this reason that I would like to suggest to the clinical reader to bear with me through the dissections and complex argumentations. Their careful scrutiny will reveal that I have indeed taken the utmost care to remain loyal to the nature of what is done and said in clinical practice. Furthermore, it is through the complex process that I present here that a new and stronger foundation for psychoanalytic dream theory is ultimately attained.

CHAPTER ONE

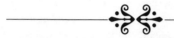

The Context: Conceptual Clarification and Previous Research

"When I use a word" Humpty Dumpty said, in rather a scornful tone "it means just what I choose it to mean—neither more nor less."

"The question is," said Alice, "whether you *can* make words mean so many different things."

"The question is," said Humpty Dumpty, "which is to be master— that's all."

Alice was too much puzzled to say anything.

—Carroll, *Through the Looking Glass*

A major role of any theory is to describe and/or explain a certain range of phenomena. Although theories also have other uses—for example, clinical applications and other practical usages—these logically rely on the way the theory understands and explains the phenomena in question. The psychoanalytic theory, for example, has been generally thought of as a theory that attempts to understand the psychic processes in the individual's mind, their interrelationships, their genetic sources, how they affect and experience behavior, and so on.

Because theories attempt to describe and explain, it follows that not any theory is just as good as any other. Although we humans may never be able to know the ultimate truth, we can nevertheless examine different theories and see which one accounts better for the data, explains better, yields better practical applications, or, in short, which theory is acceptable from the perspective of our current knowledge; or, to use the philosophical jargon, which theory is *justified*. The fact that a given theory is justified does not necessarily imply that it is true in some ultimate sense, for it may turn out upon future discoveries that it is not so. It means, however, that it is the best approximation (or is one among several equally best approximations) that is available to us at present, so that as far as we can see now there are good reasons for maintaining the theory rather than rejecting it or replacing it by another. In order for us to know that a given theory is not an arbitrary invention but a serious contender, it needs to be justified; it has to be shown to be acceptable on the basis of available data and considerations. The issue of how theories are to be justified—that is, how we know which theory is more acceptable—falls within the domain of epistemology (the study of knowledge).

These remarks on theory and justification apply, of course, to the psychoanalytic theory in general, and in particular to its dream theory, which is the subject matter of this study. If the psychoanalytic theory of dreams is to be more than an arbitrary invention that is just as good as any other, it has to be shown to be acceptable or, in other words, justified. The basic epistemological issue that underlies the psychoanalytic dream theory is, therefore: How can we justify the theory that dreams can be analyzed for their meanings in the way described by the psychoanalytic theory? And, more generally: How can we justify the claim made in psychoanalytic theory that dreams have meanings at all (rather than being mere meaningless scribbles), and that these meanings may be discovered through analysis?

These questions will be the subject matter of the present study.

PART I: CONCEPTUAL CLARIFICATION

To explore the epistemological foundation of the psychoanalytic theory of dreams requires that we first clarify some concepts that are basic to this issue. Especially important for the present discussion are the concepts of *justification* and that of *meaning*, as well as the concept of *truth*. In addition, various alternative approaches that are based on different understandings of these concepts— such as positivism, hermeneuticism, Foundationalism, Coherence theory, and the like—are also pertinent to the issue. This first chapter will focus on these topics with a twofold aim: first, to sharpen and enrich relevant concepts and ideas that are often left vague and tend to obscure important issues and distinctions; and, second, to form common ground with the reader who may be familiar with another range of concepts or with different senses of the terminology I will be using.

First, concerning the concept of *justification*, we must understand precisely what constitutes an adequate form of justification—specifically of the psychoanalytic theory—and what forms of justification have in fact been applied in the course of the development of psychoanalysis. These have been disputed topics within psychoanalysis and have suffered much from conceptual confusion. I will not attempt to conclusively resolve these very broad issues. I will rather present my formulation of them and the definitions I will be using in the course of the study, and will attempt to clarify common and potential confusions relevant to this work.

Just like the concept of justification, the concept of meaning—another highly problematic concept, both within and outside of psychoanalysis—must also be demarcated. The way in which I will be using the term and my formulations of the ways in which it has been used in the course of the development of psychoanalysis must be distinguished from numerous other formulations and usages. Here too my aim will be to provide the framework necessary for the current study. We must know what we mean by "meaning" and what Freud meant by "meaning" if we are to inquire into the possibility of obtaining these in the course of Freudian dream analysis.

There are a variety of forms of justification and many meanings to meaning. Within psychoanalysis, however, in the past twenty years the range of diversity has been truncated by a tendency to view the alternatives in terms of a spurious debate between what are portrayed as two warring camps on the field of the conceptualization of psychoanalysis—between what has been referred to as the "positivists" and the "hermeneuticists." This false debate is the product of members of the latter camp.

The psychoanalytic hermeneuticists primarily present themselves as an approach sensitive to experience and concerned with the explanation of behavior, experience, thought, and so on, in terms of meanings rather than in terms of causes, the latter relegated to the "positivistic" approach. According to the hermeneuticists, one cannot apply methods of investigation and justification that are acceptable in scientific disciplines to their experience-near meaningful explanations of the individual. The "positivistic" approach with which they contrast themselves includes all the simplistic formulations of the scientific approach to the conceptualization of psychoanalysis and consequently to its justification, and is considered to be neglectful of delicate issues of experience and meaning. This debate is spurious because matters are far from being so simple. Science has much more to offer in terms of justification and meaning (and in other respects) than is presented (or misrepresented) by the hermeneuticists. Conversely, the foundations and implications of the hermeneuticist position are problematic. The real dispute is between the broad range of conceptions that science has to offer and psychoanalytic hermeneuticism.

As I will argue, this spurious debate between "positivism" and hermeneuticism creates a false dilemma concerning the issue of justification. Justification is reduced to one of two very much simplified alternatives. The so-called "positivists" are attributed the simplistic application of natural science methods, with these methods being limited to those of an atomistic kind of Foundationalism. In contrast, the hermeneuticists tend to maintain that what testifies to the validity of the psychoanalytic endeavor are various aspects of the coherence of the patient's narrative that emerges in the clinical setting.

I will also argue that in this spurious debate the concept of meaning is similarly reduced to a very limited brand—a noncausal one. Other possible understandings of the concept are excluded and the choice facing the analyst is supposedly between the neglect of the issue of meaning or concern with this specific noncausal type.

This debate, explicitly and, more important perhaps, implicitly, pervades the psychoanalytic literature, loading many concepts with a variety of confusing connotations. Thus, in order to appreciate the definitions and formulations of "justification" and "meaning" that I will be putting forth, it will be necessary to begin with a clarification of some of this confusion. Once the false dilemma between "positivism" and hermeneuticism is clarified, the falseness of the dilemmas between meaning and cause and between atomism and coherence will also become apparent, and the place of the variety of forms of meaning and justification in psychoanalysis will be appreciated.

Here too my aim is not comprehensive exposition and resolution. Entire books have been written to this aim (e.g., Barrat, 1984; Edelson, 1988; Grünbaum, 1984, 1993; Strenger, 1991). What I hope, rather, is to create an opening in the conceptual field of psychoanalysis that would allow for the introduction of various available forms of justification into the field and for a deeper understanding of the choice between them.

"Positivism" Versus Psychoanalytic Hermeneuticism: Clarification of Their Debate and Concepts of Meaning

Since the beginning of Freud's earliest psychoanalytic writings until the present day, the question of the possibility and the status of psychoanalysis as a science has been a controversial issue. Throughout his life, Freud fought the evaluation of his theory as a "scientific fairy tale," as Krafft-Ebing already had put it way back in 1896 (Freud, 1985, p. 184; see Blass & Simon, 1992, 1994). He maintained until the end both that psychoanalysis adopts and should adopt no stance other than that of science, and that despite difficulties it was indeed successfully living up to the standards of science. More specifically, regarding the adoption of the scientific stance, and in some ways parallel to contemporary debates, Freud (1933c, p. 159) insisted that the objection that his scientific stance "overlooks the claims of the human intellect and the needs of the human mind . . . cannot be too energetically refuted." "It is," he argued, "quite without a basis, since the intellect and the mind are objects for scientific research in exactly the same way as any non-human things."

Over the years, the adversaries of Freud's scientific stance took a variety of forms. After Freud's early discussion of the scientific status of psychoanalysis, the main claim that psychoanalysis worked vigorously to refute (e.g., Hartmann, 1959; Waelder, 1960; Wallerstein, 1964) was the claim put forth by philosophers such as Hook (1959), Nagel, (1959) and Popper (1963) that Freudian psychoanalysis fails to live up to the legitimate scientific standards it set itself. But in the past thirty to forty years, the very question of whether these standards are legitimate, whether the scientific stance should be adopted, has returned to center stage—this time from within psychoanalysis itself. Gradually emerging within the metapsychology versus clinical theory debate of the 1960s and 1970s (Gill, 1976; Klein, 1976; Wallerstein, 1976), in the last two decades it has evolved into the debate over psychoanalytic hermeneuticism. While in the course of its development psychoanalytic hermeneuticism has to some degree been inspired by the discipline of philosophical hermeneutics that came into its own in the second half of this century, the present study is concerned only, and will refer only, to hermeneuticism as it has uniquely emerged within psychoanalysis.[1]

As noted earlier, the hermeneuticists focus on meaning and coherence. The way in which they focus on these issues and their stance in general has some confusing implications. This confusion is best understood through their opposition to what they consider the scientific approach to psychoanalysis. The hermeneuticists contrast their stance with that of science, but the scope of science with which they are holding a debate is, as we will soon see, very constricted and strangely defined. It is what they often coin "positivism" with which they are arguing. Accordingly, I will maintain the distinction between science on the one hand, and their term "positivism" on the other, the latter referring to the specific conception of science with which the hermeneuticists feel they are carrying on their debate.

Among the psychoanalytic hermeneuticists one may find leading psychoanalytic writers, such as Goldberg (1984), G. Klein (1976), Renik (1993, 1998), Schafer (1976, 1983), Spence (1982) in the United States, and Home (1966), Klauber (1967), Ricouer (1970, 1981), and Rycroft (1966) in Europe.[2] More impressive, however, is the infiltration of these views into everyday psychoanalytic thinking and parlance. Although I doubt that many analysts would espouse the hermeneuticist conception if its full implications were recognized and made explicit, it seems that many voice major tenets of this view when the occasion arises. It is not unusual to hear it suggested in respectable psychoanalytically oriented case presentations or lectures, by senior practitioners and beginners alike, that there is no fact of the matter regarding the patient's motives and meanings since we are not dealing with empirical reality, the domain of natural science (e.g., Haesler, 1994) or that meanings (in a psychological sense) are not really *discovered* through the psychoanalytic process but in some mysterious way come into being within the psychoanalytic session and therefore are non-causal, unlike in science (e.g., Kulka, 1994). The bottom line is that we have now recognized that psychoanalysis deals with interpretation, not with science. These are all basic tenets of the psychoanalytic hermeneuticism.

It should be noted that when such sentiments are expressed they do not always seem to be part of a comprehensive and well-formulated stance on these matters, but rather appear to be responses to local doubts and difficult questions. Questions such as how it is possible to explain the fact that analysts from different schools arrive at different understandings of the patient or how we can know for sure that the nature of the connection between certain associated ideas is indeed a causal one, may lead to a quick skepticism regarding psychoanalysis as a science and to a recourse to such hermeneuticist solutions, rather than to a more in-depth exploration of the issues. The adoption of the hermeneuticist solution is relatively easy and most practitioners do not feel compelled to devote themselves to the search for a comprehensive resolution of such philosophically oriented meta-questions. This may be because most practitioners do not encounter such questions in their ongoing clinical work. Also, it is my impression that it is believed that the answers to these questions would not have any fundamental impact on clinical work. Dealing with these philosophical issues could at best enrich the understanding of the work we are already doing. In the course of this book I hope to show otherwise; that indeed such issues do have important implications for clinical work, that for this reason the practitioner should indeed be very interested in pursuing these questions and coming to a comprehensive understanding of the issues at hand.

The Term "Positivism"

The use of the term "positivism" to refer to a natural science conception of psychoanalysis is somewhat confusing. Auguste Comte (1798–1857) had introduced the use of "positivism" to denote the view that there are general rules of methodology that apply to all fields of investigation, to the human and the natural sciences alike. However, the term does ring strange in the context of the twentieth century. Since the time of Comte, the term "positivism" has accrued new meaning, and now is usually taken as shorthand for "logical positivism." Logical positivism is a philosophical theory, introduced by what was known as the Vienna circle in the early 1920s. Influential in the first half of the twentieth century, logical positivism in its original form died in the middle of the century, with its demise becoming renowned for being the one philosophical theory to have actually been conclusively demonstrated to be false. While propounding views on all major philosophical issues from ethics to metaphysics, one of the most central theses of logical positivism is that the meaning of a proposition is its method of verification; we cannot meaningfully talk of entities other than observables (Schlick, 1959). Unobservable entities such as electrons, the unconscious, causes, and so on, are not independently existing things hidden from our view, but rather ways of describing observable data in condensed form, some even say fictions. For example, to speak about electrons is simply a short way of talking about certain observed patterns of measurements on scientific instruments. Similarly, to say that stress *causes* headache is merely to say that headache often follows stress (after all, we do not observe the causation itself, over and above the sequence of events that we observe to be following each other). In this sense, logical positivists are anti-realist with respect to unobservable, theoretical posits. (By "realism with respect to *X*" I mean, roughly speaking, as the expression is commonly used in philosophy: the belief that *X* is "not merely in our minds" so to speak; that it has a reality that is independent of people's thoughts about it.)

There are certain aspects of logical positivism that Freud may seem to have espoused. However, many aspects of logical positivism are plainly irrelevant to Freud's work; regarding many others the relationship is unclear, and their anti-realist perspective clearly runs counter to the blatant realism that (for the most part) pervades Freud's writings. Freud was convinced that his work led him to discover realities that lay beyond the directly observed data. Strangely, those who label Freud a positivist do not regard his realism to be contradictory to his alleged positivism, but rather as further evidence of it (Hoffmann, 1991; Schafer, 1983, p. 184). Conversely, those eschewing metapsychology, and even the reality of causation on the ground that these are not observable, consider themselves to be moving away from this positivistic trend (Home, 1966; Klein, 1976; Schafer, 1976). This unfortunate choice of terminology is not only one of the sources of the confusion that arises in the application of the term "positivism" within psychoanalysis. This choice also encourages the dismissal of the scientific approach to psychoanalysis on the grounds that the time has finally come to lay it to rest: "positivism" has died. Now to some other sources of confusion.

The Hermeneuticist Critique of Positivism

The scientific view, according to the hermeneuticist formulation, is concerned with objective facts and with causes. While those holding a scientific view may agree with this, it is the hermeneuticist definitions of the terms *fact* and *cause* that make matters highly problematic. Two major problems lie at the heart of the matter: First, they define cause and psychic facts in such a way that the two cannot belong to the same domain; and, second, they define meaning in such a way that the search for it, by the mere force of definition, cannot have anything to do with the observation of facts and the determining of causal connections. Let us turn to the details of their critique.

The First Critique of Positivism: Psychic States Cannot be Discussed in Terms of Causation. This position has several (partially overlapping) versions including the following.

a. Accessibility of psychic states. Psychic states are either not accessible to the observer or are contaminated by the subjectivity of the observer, his or her theories and methods, so that we can never really know the fact of the matter regarding these states. As Roy Schafer explains (1976, p. 205): "We psychoanalysts cannot rightly claim to establish causality through our investigations in any rigorous and untrivial sense of the term. Control, production, mathematical precision are beyond our reach, for we are not engaged in the kind of investigation that can yield these results." Also in psychoanalytic investigations, according to Schafer, in contrast to "all other fields of inquiry, there can be no theory-free and method-free facts" (Schafer, 1983, p. 188). Consequently we do not have access to the psychic states themselves. Rather "all perception is interpretation in context" (Schafer, 1983, p. 184). Or as Renik (1993, 1998) explains, in the analytic situation "subjectivity is irreducible," meaning that the analyst's clinical observations of the patient's psychical states are no more than constructions determined by the analyst's personal subjective experiences and interests. What follows is that there is no point in talking of the causation of such states.

b. Non-factuality of psychic states. Psychic states have a unique status such that there is no real fact of the matter regarding them. Those who maintain this position often make much use of Freud's ill-chosen term "material reality," which he contrasts with "psychical reality." While Freud used the term to distinguish between reality and fantasy, hermeneuticists have portrayed the distinction as being between events that have real existence and psychical events, which do not (Ricouer, 1981, p. 254). In line with this view Ricouer (1974, p. 186) contends, for example, that "there are no 'facts' in psychoanalysis, but rather the interpretation of a narrated history." Others have associated this nonfactual view with the notion that subjective states spontaneously come into being, especially in the course of analytic treatment (Home, 1966, p. 45; Schafer, 1978, pp. 48–49). Or as Hanly (1990) in a sharp critique has referred to it: the notion that there is an "intrinsic indefiniteness of the human mind which allows it to slip away from any description that would seek to correspond with some fixed and determinate nature" (p. 376). In any case, since according to this view there is no fact of the matter regarding these psychic states, here too the consequence is that they are beyond causation.

c. *Causation does not apply to psychic events.* Causation belongs only to the domain of material events; hence, psychic events are not causal. Here there are two versions, one that we can talk of human causation only on a neurological level (e.g., Basch, 1976, pp. 72–73); the other and more common version is that we can talk of causation only in terms of the effects of real external events on the person (e.g., Rycroft, 1966, p. 16; Schafer, 1976). The neurological processes underlying our psychic states are part of a causal network as are our nonpsychic observable behaviors. In other words, real observable past events causally effect present ones; thus, for example, our present character traits may be causally determined by events that actually occurred in childhood. But psychic reality, our fantasies, wishes, intentions, and so on, lack the physical substance necessary for causation. Once we reject the reduction of the psychic to the biological, and put aside knowledge regarding external reality and its influence of past events, there is no longer any room to talk of causation. "The ideas of causes has a place only in the behavioristic approach to people" (Schafer, 1976, p. 370). An auxiliary component of this view is that intentions, reasons, wishes, and dispositions are not considered to be causes. These are personal constructs of noncausal status (Klein, 1976, p. 43; Schafer, 1976, pp. 204–205. This position has been discussed at length by Grünbaum, 1984, and Strenger, 1991).

The Second Critique of Positivism: Observation and Causation are Divorced from the Search for Meaning. This is a most central point and, as will later be seen, is of great significance to the issue of psychoanalytic dream interpretation. The "positivists" are said to be involved in some kind of scientific endeavor *rather than* devoting themselves to the study of meaning. This in part follows from the unusual definition of causation and the hermeneuticist view of the epistemic difficulties regarding the knowledge of psychic states (see the previous section on accessibility). More specifically, since causation is allegedly a category that applies only to biology and external nonpersonal events, the "positivists," who are concerned with causation, cannot be concerned with meaning per se. Also, since the recognition of psychic states is essential to elaboration of meaning, "positivists," who apply objective methods, which cannot perceive these states, cannot really elaborate meaning. As Home (1966) affirms: "Because meaning is an aspect of the living subject known to us through identification it cannot be investigated by the methods and logic of science for these are applicable only to the dead object, or to the object perceived as dead" (p. 47).

But the disjunction of meaning and causation extends beyond this. There appears to be an argument to the effect that even if we assume that causation is applicable to psychic states, and even if we assume that these states may be observed, the search for meaning is simply inherently unrelated to the search for causes. Meaning, in any sense relevant to psychoanalysis, is noncausal. In this context Freud's concern with meaning is often contrasted with his desire to arrive at a causal understanding. For example, Basch (1976, p. 73) writes that "Freud was to assert many times . . . that psychoanalysts are concerned with meaning alone, only to then immediately try to hypothesize causal explanations for the events termed meaningful." In a similar but more extreme vein Home (1966, p. 43) writes that "In discovering that the symptom had meaning and that basing his treatment on this hypothesis, Freud took the psychoanalytic study of neurosis out of the world of science into the world of the humanities, because a meaning is not the product of causes but the creation of a subject."

Taking into account these definitions of mental states, causes, and meaning, "positivism" emerges as an irrelevant and misguided endeavor within the psychoanalytic setting. It tries to establish facts to the neglect of the epistemic impossibility resulting from the contamination of the data by theory; it seeks causation where there is none or where it cannot be determined; and it is involved with the effects of external reality and biology, rather than with the intrapsychic world of the individual. The positivistic concern with psychic reality is not a concern with subjectivity or with meaning.

A Response to the Hermeneuticist Critique of Positivism: Psychic States Can be Discussed in Terms of Causation

The confusion that underlies the hermeneuticist conclusions and their premises regarding subjectivity, causation, meaning, and so on, that are at its base is quite extensive and a comprehensive study of it would take us way too far afield. In this section I will briefly respond to their first critique—that psychic states cannot be discussed in terms of causation. A response to their second critique, which focuses on their claim that observation and causation are not related to a search for meaning, requires a broader statement on meaning and its relationship to causation. I will discuss this broader point in the following section, and in that context I will address the hermeneuticist critique.

a. *Response to the argument against accessibility of psychic states.* First, it should be noted that anyone working within the field of psychoanalysis must presuppose that the psychoanalyst has some access to the patient's psychic states, particularly to the suffering for which he or she seeks help. To the extent that we take psychic states to be the subject matter of our interest in the psychoanalytic setting, we are thereby assuming that they are accessible to the observer. To what are we responding in the patient if we have no idea about his or her subjective mental states? What is it we are understanding, if psychic states are not accessible?

Furthermore, the fact that a given psychic state is "subjective" in the sense of being inside the person and hidden from *direct* view does in no way imply that it is impossible to assess its existence in some indirect way. Indeed, this is precisely what science does: It studies phenomena that are not directly observable—and with a tremendous degree of success. Electrons, black holes, electric currents, the evolution and disappearance of ancient species, the birth of stars, are no more observable than unconscious desires or hidden traumas. Scientists can directly observe only remote by-products of these phenomena, and even those usually only through the mediation of readings on their instruments. But this hardly shows that they have no access to such phenomena. In a similar way, there is every reason to believe that through the person's behavior, gestures, self-description, and so on, we can in principle learn about his or her psychic world.

In fact, this is what we commonly do in everyday interactions with others. By attending to other people's behavior and words, we commonly learn about their headaches, thoughts, anxieties, or worries—though, like all facts, not with complete certainty. In this respect we are like scientists who attend to the language and behavior of earthquakes, tissues in test tubes, or light from distant stars, and uncover the hidden geological, biological, or astronomical reality that they express. Thus, the direct unobservability of psychic states in no way implies their inaccessibility. To deny a priori our accessibility to them just because they are subjective and thus hidden from view is to reject the whole of science with a prescientific naiveté.

The claim that the involvement of the observer, with his or her theories and methods, bars access to psychic states is equally untenable. Admittedly, it is possible to maintain that our theoretical precommitments and our methods influence the way we perceive the facts. Whatever we observe in our patients and whatever our patients tell us are already "colored" by the observer's conceptual scheme or way of looking at the world. That something must be wrong with this argument is clear, however, from the fact that it can be applied not just to psychic facts but also to every single aspect of our world. Our theoretical precommitments and conceptual scheme should "color" not only psychic data but chemical, biological, meteorological, and everyday facts just as well. Hence, if the argument were sound, we would not have access to facts in any scientific field. It would seem, however, that the hermeneuticists do not wish to maintain that there are no facts accessible to science at all, but rather only that psychoanalytic facts are inaccessible, but the basis for this distinction remains obscure.[3] Moreover, it is important to recognize that even if the world can be seen only through our theories, this does not mean that we do not have access to it. The possible theory-ladenness of the facts that we encounter merely implies that we can know only of the world as it made known to us through our human conceptual schemes. This is true in the realm of physics and psychoanalysis alike.

   b. *Response to the argument against factuality of psychic states.* The idea that the domain of the "psychic" is not factual, that there is no fact of the matter concerning "psychic" states, sounds rather incredible already at first glance. Do the hermeneuticists seriously wish to maintain that there is no fact of the matter as to whether or not I am experiencing distress? Do they wish to claim that it is neither true nor false that my patient has, say, a longing for a father figure? That, more specifically, whether or not she has such longing is not just unknowable but in fact neither true nor false; not in the sense that the situation is a borderline case between yes and no (as dusk is neither really day nor really night), but in the sense that it is purely and completely a matter of interpretation? It is hard to imagine what this can possibly mean. We may assume that hermeneuticists would agree that there is a fact of the matter regarding whether I am now sitting and writing this book. Were they to claim otherwise it would be very strange. Why then should there be no fact of the matter regarding subjective states?

Hermeneuticists are likely to object that writing a book is objective while psychic states are subjective. But here one should wonder whether they have not been misled by some mystical halo of the term "subjective." In its original use, "subjective" simply means to exist within the subject. It is a geographical term, so to speak, that assigns to anxieties and pains a location inside the person, in contrast to books and chairs that are located outside the subject, in the domain of objects, the "objective" realm. Obviously, the fact that something happens to reside within the subject does not imply, at least not by itself, that there is no matter of fact about it. But here "subjective" has become synonymous with "ephemeral" or "hazy," denoting the twilight zone between reality and fiction, and contrasted with facts.

One common argument designed to show that there are no psychic matters of fact is once again based on the fact that we have no data about the psychic life that is theory-free. Here the earlier argument is taken one step further. It is now claimed that if all that we observe is "colored" by our theoretical precommitments and our methods, then it is not that facts are inaccessible (as claimed in that earlier argument) but rather that there are no facts, only interpretations. But here too the weakness of this argument becomes immediately apparent when it is recognized that it can be applied not only to psychic facts but to all facts. If the argument is sound, it should take away the factual basis not only from psychoanalysis but from all of science.

We must, therefore, conclude that if psychic states are in some ultimate sense not hard facts, they are still in the same domain as scientific facts, and hence are sufficiently hard for scientific investigation of the type commonly carried out in standard science. The point is that even if the world in which we find ourselves is a human interpretation, it still contains elements—such as the chemical structure of water or the etiology of anxiety—that we cannot reinterpret and modify at will, so that there is a definite fact of the matter about them (as they are within the human world). Similarly, there are facts about the nature of the fantasies and feelings passing through a patient's mind. Even if our world is a human interpretation, even if it is God's dream, it contains elements that are one way rather than another, which is to say, facts, or if you wish: facts-within-our-human-world.

The claim that psychic states are nonfactual ultimately emerges as strange, and the arguments in its favor obscure. Careful study of the way this claim is put forth and discussed suggests that a possible explanation of the obscurity may lie in the neglect of the distinction between a content—an idea in itself (e.g., the number 7, the concept of motherhood, or specifically of one's mother) and the state of *having the content*, possessing the idea; for example, between the idea of mother and a fantasy whose content is mother. Contents—of thoughts, desires, fantasies, and so on—may be abstract. They may refer to nonmaterial objects (e.g., as in a thought about the number 7) or to material objects that are either real (e.g., as in a desire to have a horse) or unreal (e.g., as in a fantasy about a unicorn), to objects clearly defined or to indeterminate objects. In contrast to the abstract contents, the *having* of the content is a real psychic event.

If one neglects this distinction, one may treat psychic events as unreal just because their contents are unreal. From the realization that unicorns are not factual, one may conclude that fantasies about unicorns are not factual. But this move is obviously fallacious. There are perhaps no facts about unicorns, but there are facts about the patient's *fantasy about* unicorns: It is a recurring event that started at a certain point in time and exerts various influences on the patient's behavior and thoughts. Although contents of psychic states need not be real, the psychic states themselves are real; they are in a person's mind, and as such there is a fact of the matter regarding them. I may have a fantasy that my mother had always hit me as a child. This may be completely untrue. The fantasy, however, as the presence of the idea in my head, exists. There is a fact of the matter regarding it. It is a real state. It is real even if the content to which it refers may not yet be clearly formed or clear, or if it refers only to some kind of vague potential. This would simply mean that my psychic event, or fantasy—which is as real as any real event in our world—has distorted, unformed, unclear, fuzzy, or vague contents.

One may perhaps object that in cases of fuzzy or vague psychic states it is not the content that is fuzzy but rather the psychic state itself. But even if this were true, it still would not make the having of the content any less real. The fact that a painting or a cloud is fuzzy does not mean that its reality is in question. Even vague psychic states are real and factual.

c. *Response to the argument that causation does not apply to psychic states.* Causation does indeed apply to psychic events. In some limited sense, the question of causation in the psychic domain may be considered as a matter of definition. Someone could arbitrarily decide to define causation in a way that delimits it to biological entities, or in a way that makes it applicable only to the effects of real external events. One could also define it such that it would relate only to interstellar influences. To do this, however, would be strange and would miss the point. Why should the concept of causation be limited in this way? Causation means, very simply, "bringing about." To say that an anxiety caused a fantasy is simply to say that the anxiety brought about, or gave birth to, the fantasy. It is hard to see what is wrong with such a formulation. Consider, for instance, the idea, held by some, that causation should be applied only to the effects of external reality. Why, for example, should the term causation be considered applicable only in the study of how the *real* mother affected the psychic state of her son and not how an *idea* the son has about his mother (regardless of its relationship to reality) affects his psychic state? If we adopt a common analysis from the field of philosophy, we may say, roughly speaking, that to say that *A* caused *B* is to say that *A* was followed by *B*, and were *A* not to occur, *B* would not have occurred either. Clearly, according to this common and commonsensical conception of causation, one psychic event may be the cause of another psychic event, in the sense that the former was necessary for the second to happen.

Is it because psychic events are considered less real than other events that they are excluded from having a causal status? As we have seen, the fact that we do not see our psychic events, the fact that the contents of the psychic events are abstract, does not make the psychic state of *having* the contents any less real. And yet in the literature it appears as if the deepening of Freud's early recognition that we are not dealing with historical truth, but rather with psychic reality, removes causation from the picture. That is, it is as if once we acknowledge that in the clinical setting we cannot assuredly reconstruct the childhood events that determine the patient's current predicament, our interpretations no longer deal with real entities, regarding which there are indeed questions of what determined what. It would seem that this position has recently become so deeply ingrained in psychoanalysis that some version of it even infiltrates into the writings and case studies of analytic thinkers who acknowledge that the role of causation has been too readily dismissed by the hermeneuticists (see Strenger, 1991, pp. 58, 73).

The arguments in favor of psychic events being causal are quite plain. Psychic events (e.g., thinking, believing, fantasizing, feeling, etc.) are real events that occur at a particular time. As such, they are, like all other real events that take place in real time, subject to causation: They influence, are influenced, bring about, and are brought about by other events. This is especially obvious if one is a materialist and does not believe in a nonmaterial soul, for then one should agree that psychic events take place in our brain and as such are subject to causation.

Furthermore, whether one believes that psychic events are in the brain or in the soul, there are simple cases in which it is obvious that these events cause and are caused. Think what it would mean to deny this. For example, the state of distress causes (brings about, gives birth to) the expression of pain. Insult causes distress. Clearly, it is not just a coincidence that one event tends to follow the other. Were we to assume otherwise, a patient could cry in pain but we would have no reason to believe that the cry is a result of (i.e., was caused by) her actually being in a state of distress, for this would involve the attribution of causation to that state. We could not assume that the insult, or any other distress-correlated event, such as falling on one's face, actually brought on the distress. So whether distress (or any other mental event) is a material brain-event or a nonmaterial soul-event, either way the correlation clearly shows that it is subject to causal relations.

Do the hermeneuticists wish to deny these obvious cases of causation? I would gather that many of those who reject the "positivistic" position do not opt for this alternative. Rather, they refer to the relationships that I call (in accordance with common use) "causes" in different terms such as, motives, wishes, intentions, and dispositions, which are said to "bring about," "be responsible for," "give birth to," or similar expressions, which are merely different ways of speaking of causation. The only advantage of not referring to these as "causes" is that in this way they are supposedly no longer subject to the scientific standards to which causation is subject. It is as if a new and wholly other standard must be applied when we come to the domain of persons and psychic reality.

In sum, the arguments put forth here show that the hermeneuticists' claim that mental states cannot be discussed in terms of causal processes is untenable. Their first main critique is found to be misguided. In the next section, in which we examine the concept of meaning, their second critique of science as irrelevant to the psychoanalytic interest with meaning emerges as equally untenable.

Meaning and Causation

The concept of meaning has many different meanings and applications in different fields. What it refers to is not something to be discovered or assumed, but is rather a matter of definition. The lack of recognition of this transforms matter of definition into matters of self-evident givens and results in spurious dispute. Examples of this may be found in the accusation that Freud put aside his concern with meaning to address questions of causation (e.g., Basch, 1976), or that he mistakenly assumed that meaning was tied to causation (e.g., Stolorow & Atwood, 1982). In Freud's terms, however, it is not possible to put aside meaning for causation, nor for him could meaning be mistakenly assumed to be tied to causation. For Freud meaning was *defined* by its tie to causation. Those who accuse him of neglect or mistake define meaning differently. As a rule, it would seem that in the psychoanalytic literature the referent of the term "meaning" is taken for granted, although different analysts are in fact referring to different things by the term. The result of this is not only misguided claims of neglect and mistake, but also a large degree of obscurity. To clarify matters, let us make two basic distinctions.

Two Distinctions Regarding Meaning.

a. *Meaning within the subject versus meaning to an observer:* An expressed content can be attended to in two basic ways. One can wonder what the subject expressing the content is expressing. What does he mean? This is the "meaning within the subject." On the other hand, one can wonder what the content being expressed by the subject means to me the observer. This is the meaning to the observer. In the one, the content is determined in terms of the subject's psychic context, and in the other in terms of the psychic context of the observer. For example, when the subject says he feels hungry, we may be concerned with what he is expressing in this statement; what he means by it. Alternately we may be concerned with what this expression means to me. In terms of *my* psychic context it may be that an expression of hunger means an egocentric focus on bodily needs. This is what it means to me. But, of course, it may have nothing whatsoever to do with the meaning within the subject. In fact, he may be hungry because he is fasting out of identification with the starving people of India. There may, at times, be much more confluence between what things mean to the subject and what they mean to the observer. Empathic understanding is based on such confluence. The observer may know what the subject is meaning because given such confluence there will be some similarity between what an expression means both to the observer and within the subject. At other times, there may be meaning to the observer while there is none in terms of the subject or even when there is no subject. This is the case when one reacts to a Rorschach card (although the observer may transform the task to what the alleged subject who created the Rorschach card wished to express).

Of course, there is also the option that a person take an observer stance in relation to oneself. In this case she would wonder, from the third-person perspective, what she had said means to herself.

This distinction between meaning within the subject of a certain individual and meaning to the observer of that some individual usually goes unnoted (Peterfreund [1971] is an exception). The impact of this becomes most apparent when it comes to dream interpretation. To understand the meaning of a dream may mean either to understand its meaning within the subject who expressed it at the time of the dream, or to understand what it means to the dreamer, as observer, when awake. As we will see, it is not self-evident that the two are one and the same, and which of the two is being referred to is not always clear.

In what follows I continue with the elaboration of the meaning within the subject.

b. *The meaning of a statement versus the meaning of stating.* This distinction is between the meaning of the content being expressed and the meaning of the act of stating or expressing the content. For example, if a person suddenly says, "I *really* love my mother," I can wonder what is the meaning (within the subject) of the statement. Depending on the person, the context, as well as on one's theory of meaning, this statement can have various meanings. One possible meaning is that the person has a feeling of love for her mother. Another possible meaning is that she actually hates her mother and this statement is a concealed expression of this. There are, of course, many other possible ways that this statement could be understood. Alternatively, however, the question may be not what she means, but what is the meaning of the fact that she is making this statement. Perhaps she had heard or thought something that made her feel guilty toward her mother and this caused her to state what she did. Or it may have been that someone she admired just said these words and she wished to emulate her, and so on. Here the act of stating means, "I feel guilty," or "I wish to be just like my admired friend." As we will later see, according to some formulations the meaning of stating is considered to be part of the meaning of the statement. In this case, the meaning of the statement would include, for example, both the feeling of love and the feeling of guilt.

The distinctions that we have discussed thus far may be charted as follows (Figure 1.1):

Figure 1.1. Meaning Distinctions Chart

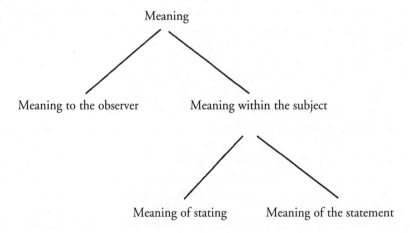

Meaning of the Statement: "Described," "Created," and "Discovered" Meanings. When we speak of meaning we are speaking of a relationship between two entities. We say that X means Y. To understand the meaning of meaning in psychoanalysis we must define what these entities are and the nature of the relationship between them. Within psychoanalysis we may distinguish between three broad categories of "meaning" that differ on this latter dimension.

To clarify matters, let us return to the distinction just made between a *content*, which is abstract, and the *having of the content*, which is a real and concrete psychic event or state. It is possible to speak of meaning in terms of relationships between contents. Relationships between entities of this kind are found, for example, in semantics. When we speak of the meaning of the concept of "happiness" we are speaking of the relationship between this content and another content, for example: "Happiness" means joy or pleasure. The relationship in this instance is one of convention. There are other forms of relationship between contents, which refer to other senses of the term meaning. For example, we may inquire into the meaning of "happiness" in a philosophical sense. Here too we would be relating to contents, abstract ideas, but the relationship would be conceptual, as when Aristotle defines the meaning of happiness as an activity of the soul in accordance with excellence (Aristotle, 1963).

In contrast, we can also talk of meaning in terms of the relationship between one psychic event or state and another psychic event or state (each one of which may have various contents).[4] For example, when we want to know the meaning of happiness in psychoanalysis we want to know the meaning, not of the abstract concept of happiness, but of the actual psychic event of happiness or, in other words, the meaning of being in the state of happiness. A satisfactory account of such meaning would refer to other psychic states. For example, we may say that happiness means to the individual the feeling of being admired by a significant person, or the idea of having fulfilled an Oedipal wish. Here we identified meaning as the connection between two psychic states: e.g., the state of happiness and the feeling of being admired.

Note that in this example meaning is portrayed as a *general* connection between one *type* of psychic states (states of happiness) to another type (feelings of being admired). Meaning as a general connection between types of states can be found in general theories, as in the case of Freud's theories regarding the meaning of anxiety, the meaning of jealousy, and, as we will see, the meaning of the dream. Against the background of such general theories, we may also speak of meaning as a *specific* connection in a *particular* individual between one specific psychic event or state to another. Thus, we may inquire into the meaning of happiness in a general and theoretical way, or alternatively we may be concerned with the meaning of happiness in one specific person, that is, in terms of an individual's personal context of meaning. It is the latter that is of interest to us here.

So far we have isolated the general sense in which we speak of meaning in psychoanalysis, and identified it with connections between psychic entities, either general types of entities or particular ones. However, the issue now is: What kind of connections are such meaning-connections? The answer is that embedded in the psychoanalytic literature are three different psychoanalytic approaches to the nature of these connections. We may, therefore, speak of three different categories of meaning within psychoanalysis. I will refer to these three categories as "*meaning described*," "*meaning created*," and "*meaning discovered*." Each of these is based on a different conception of the nature of meaning-connections between psychic events. "Meaning described" refers to an experiential relationship, "meaning created" to a thematic (i.e., semantic, or content-based) relationship, and "meaning discovered" to a causal relationship.

More specifically, when we speak of X meaning Y for a certain subject, we may be referring to three alternative connections between X and Y. First, we may be referring to the fact that the subject has *an experience* of X being tied to Y. For example, a person may feel that his happiness is tied to his feeling of being admired by a significant person.[5] This feeling may be mistaken in the sense that it does not reflect his inner reality. He may be completely happy independently of any admiration, but his experience creates the tie between these psychic events. If we are interested in meaning in this sense, what we need to do is to carefully read the descriptions offered by the subject. Our question here would be how the individual experiences or describes the connections between his various psychic entities, not how they really are connected. Hence I refer to this form of meaning as "*meaning described*." It should be stressed that what characterizes this approach is not the claim that attunement to experience is important for determining meaning. All psychoanalytic approaches would agree on that. Rather what characterizes this approach is the claim that meanings are *determined* by the description of the experience. Meaning *is* the immediate experience of connections between psychic entities, the way a certain psychic entity "is embedded in the ongoing course of . . . experiencing" (Atwood & Stolorow, 1984, p. 99).

Analysts who maintain this descriptive view of meaning often do not do so exclusively. They usually do not make do with the meanings that the individual describes, but rather consider there to be additional meanings that in due course should become experientially available. To relate to these additional meaning it is necessary to rely on one of the other two psychoanalytic views of meaning to which I now turn.

One alternate sense in which we may speak of X meaning Y would refer to a *thematic* tie between these psychic events, that is, the connection between their themes, or contents. Thus, when we speak of X meaning Y for a certain subject we may be saying that there is a common theme between what one psychic event (X) is about and what another psychic event (Y) is about, regardless of whether the two are related in any other sense. For example, within a specific individual there may exist a thematic tie between happiness and admiration based on the common theme of worthwhileness. This individual feels happiness to be a worthwhile state, and he also feels being admired to be a worthwhile state. To sharpen the point, let us assume that in fact there is no psychological connection between the two states of worthwhileness; the two have developed in him independently of each other. Nevertheless, there is within this individual a meaning-connection between happiness and admiration—that is, a common theme between the content "happiness is worthwhile" and "being admired is worthwhile"—even though there is no psychological connection between the two. Here the meaning is not necessarily immediately felt or experienced, nor does it reflect some internal connection in the psyche of the subject. Rather, it reflects a semantic connection between two ideas, one that may be formulated (either by the subject or by another observer) through a literary analysis of the contents. Of course, the subject may happen to experience that thematic connection, but the point is that it is not the experience that constitutes the connection.

Meaning as thematic connections is not read off the subject's experience, nor is it discovered to exist inside the subject's psyche or experiences in any way. It is rather woven, so to speak, between the subject's statements regarding his psychic entities, and added on to what is already found within him. In a sense, speaking of thematic connections between a person's statements is similar to writing a story, which connects the different statements into a coherent script. Meaning based on this kind of connections can therefore be seen as a literary creation of the observer—whether the subject observing himself or another person. I will therefore call it *"meaning created."* This view of meaning is central to all psychoanalytic hermeneuticists, but perhaps has been most forcefully presented by Schafer (1983) in his focus on the analyst's function of creating stories and by Spence (1982a, 1982b), who speaks of the analyst's function as a "pattern-maker" rather than a "pattern finder."

The third sense in which we may speak of X meaning Y refers to a *causal* connection between the two psychic events. Thus, when we say that X means Y we mean that in some way Y brought about X or influenced the way in which it appeared. This connection does not have to be experienced in order to exist, nor does there necessarily have to be a thematic tie between the two (although in psychoanalysis there usually is). In our example of "happiness" this would mean that the feeling of happiness and the feeling of being admired would be *causally* attached to each other, they would be part of the same causal network, rather than attached merely by after-the-fact experience or thematic interpretation. Since this category of meaning is based on a relationship that does indeed reflect a reality—that is, an inner reality, or actual causal ties between psychic events—meaning in this sense is something to discover, not to postulate or create. We may, therefore, refer to this category as *"meaning discovered."* This approach to meaning is the classical one and has dominated psychoanalysis since the time of Freud until the emergence of psychoanalytical hermeneuticism in recent years (see Friedman, 1996, p. 261).

It may be noted that in all three categories we are talking about the meaning of contents that exist in the mind, not about abstract contents, but only in "meaning discovered" is the meaning itself something that exists in the mind. That is, only in "meaning discovered" is the *relationship* between the psychic entities that exist in the mind, something that also actually exists in the mind.

It may also be noted that "meaning discovered" resembles "meaning created" in that in both meaning is determined from a third-person perspective (even if it is a subject's own third-person observation on herself). In contrast, in "meaning experienced" meaning is based on a first-person perspective; it is based on the subject's immediate experience. More important, however, the following distinction between "meaning discovered" and the other two categories should be noted: "Meaning discovered" refers to a causal relationship between psychic events while the other two kinds of meaning refer to noncausal relationships. Before further exploring this distinction and the nature of the relationship between meaning and causation, let us first glance at one more example through which the differences between the categories of meaning become apparent.

Example: "The meaning of Jane's fear of headaches is guilt."

In this sentence, meaning is specified as a relationship or connection between the psychic event of fear of headaches and the psychic event of feelings of guilt. From the perspective of "meaning described," the relationship would be experiential. She *feels* a tie between the two. The meaning would be arrived at by attending to Jane's description of her experience of a connection between her fear of headaches and her sense of guilt. For example, she may say that she feels that the fear appears whenever she feels that she should be reprimanded for not having lived up to what she should have.

From the perspective of "meaning created," the relationship between the fear and the guilt would be thematic. Through a simple analysis of abstract ideas we can readily see that the concept of guilt implies deserving punishment, and that the concept of punishment implies suffering such as pain (headaches). Thus, the guilt ties in well, in a literary sense, with the fear of headache and establishes a thematic connection with it. Meaning here would be arrived at by observing thematic ties between the fear of headaches and the sense of guilt. Coherence between the two ideas would be sought. For example, one possible scenario is that in the course of the analytic sessions Jane speaks of the untimely death of her mother years ago due to a sudden blood clot. She also expresses her feeling of her intellectual superiority over her mother, and the feeling that the expression of the superiority can kill. One may then point to a connection between the idea expressed in the fear of being hurt in the brain (the headache) and the idea expressed in the fear of hurting the brain (causing the blood clot) because of the brain (her intellectual superiority). Similarly, guilt—which is what Jane feels—can be tied to the idea of a retributive system based on a combination of "an eye for an eye" and "cut off the arm that steals." In this way, we may tie the guilt that Jane feels with the idea that one should be hurt in the way that one hurt others and in a way that should prevent the possibility of future hurt. We may then point to the parallel between the fear of headaches and its associated ideas and the guilt and its associated ideas. The idea of guilt, as expressed in Jane's feelings, has the same pattern as does her fear of headaches. One may understand the fear of headaches in terms of guilt. In this sense the fear means guilt.

It is important to emphasize that if we are interested only in "meaning created," then we should not be concerned with the issue of whether or not the above fear–guilt thematic connection reflects Jane's actual psychology. As far as we are concerned, Jane's fear and her guilt may be completely unrelated in terms of her inner psychology. Each one of the two may have developed independently of the other. If it is only the "literary," thematic connection in which we are interested, then this possibility should not bother us (perhaps because we would argue that it makes no sense to try to discover causal psychological facts). We would be only concerned with weaving a coherent story, that will bring together the themes expressed in her various feelings.

From the perspective of "meaning discovered" the relationship between the fear of headaches and the guilt would be causal. It would be guilt that in some way effected the appearance of the fear of headaches. (As we will later see, the nature of the causal connection may take different forms, not necessarily only the simple one of direct causation). Here too attention would be given to the context and to thematic relations, as well as to her subjective descriptions, but the focus would be on how the fear brings about the guilt, or actually finds expression through it. Someone interested in this kind of meaning would want to know whether indeed Jane is feeling guilty and whether there is indeed a latent connection in her mind between the headache and the guilt. Did "guilt" bring on or did it not bring on Jane's specific flow of ideas related to the fear of headaches? From this perspective, only if it did, only if there were a causal connection such that the fear of headaches becomes a vehicle for the guilt, could we speak of the meaning of the fear in terms of guilt. A thematic connection would not suffice and Jane's own descriptions of feeling that there is a connection would be enlightening, but would not in themselves directly tell us of such a connection.

Given these different kinds of meanings, one may proceed to ask: What is Jane supposed to understand from the fact that it has just been suggested to her by her analyst that one meaning of her fear of headaches is guilt? The answer is, perhaps, that it would depend on how things were said. If it were said in a way that emphasized that this is her experience or—although an unlikely statement within the analytic setting—that one may see an interesting literary connection between the fear and the guilt, then perhaps she would accept this suggestion as referring to meaning on these levels. But in the absence of such a special emphasis, Jane may be inclined to understand the suggestion as referring to "meaning discovered." In this case she would conclude that her analyst is speaking of a possible causal connection between her feelings of guilt and her fear of headaches. In my experience this kind of understanding of meaning is the most common. In interpreting personal matters most people want to know what is really going on in their psyche and think that they are talking about an actual or true state of affairs. When told that something means something, most people take this to mean that it "*really* means" this, not that there is an experience of it meaning this, or that there is the possibility of creating such a meaning. When people inquire into the meaning of their mental states they want to know what those states are doing there. "What does it mean that I fear headaches" for many is interchangeable with "Why do I fear headaches" and the kind of answer that is sought is a real one; real, not necessarily in the sense of an external reality (e.g., "Because as a child I had hurt my mother—actually"), but real in the sense of causal internal psychic states (e.g., "Because of my sense of guilt").

To make a little further use of this example we may return to the distinction, mentioned earlier, between *meaning of the statement* and the *meaning of stating*. Up until now we have focused on the meaning of Jane's statement regarding her fear. But why is she telling us of it now? This is the meaning of stating. There may be many causes of this (which extend beyond what would be perhaps her overt reason of wanting to express what it is she believes that she is expressing). Something may have reminded her of her fear, some repressing factor may have just been overcome, and so on. We may try to isolate further some specific cause. For example, it may be that Jane suddenly recognized that her fear of headaches had begun to diminish, that she was "getting better," and that the consequence would be that she would have to end her analysis. Being attached to her analyst, this was something she wished to avoid. In this context, the stating of her fear of headaches could be seen to be an expression regarding how "sick" she still is. Since the distinction between the meaning of stating and the meaning of the statement is not explicit in psychoanalysis, many analysts (Freud included) relate to both kinds of meaning under one heading. Thus they would say that Jane's latent expression of sickness—the cause and meaning of her stating (and feeling) her fear of headaches at this point—is one of the meanings of her statement regarding her fear of headaches.

Meaning and Causation in the Light of the Framework for Meaning. A Response to the Hermeneuticist Claim that Causation Is Divorced from the Search for Meaning. Now that we have made the threefold distinction between "meaning described," "meaning created," and "meaning discovered," we may take another look at the relationship between meaning and causation in psychoanalysis. This will provide the response to the hermeneuticists' second critique of science, namely, that its focus on causation renders it irrelevant to the psychoanalytic aim that focuses on a search for meaning. Two points here are central.

(1) *There is no contradiction between a concern with meaning and a concern with causation.* As we have seen, what meaning refers to in psychoanalysis

is in part a matter of definition. The three different psychoanalytic senses of meaning refer to three different phenomena. One can, as do the hermeneuticists, choose to define meaning only in the first or second sense, rejecting the notion of "meaning discovered," and thus exclude causal connections from the domain of meanings by the sheer force of a narrowed definition. But this would simply express the fact that one decided, rather arbitrarily, not to capture all the senses of the term and to leave out "meaning discovered." It would be analogous to deciding to define "a dog" as not taller than one meter, and thus to separate Great Danes from other dogs by the sheer force of this arbitrary definition. Surely there is a sense in which meaning and causation are intimately tied.

A hermeneuticist who is interested merely in "meaning described" or "meaning created" might argue at this point that the causal notion of meaning, namely "meaning discovered," expresses disregard for the noncausal senses of the term. Such an argument, however, would be without basis. Someone who is interested in "meaning discovered" is not interested in blind causation, but also in subjective experiences, their contents and themes. An inquiry into meaning discovered does not focus solely on statements that A caused B, since, as was noted in the previous example, in order to understand the causal meaning of, say, fear, it is necessary to attend to experiences and themes. Of course, someone who is concerned with "meaning discovered" would not view the other, noncausal kinds of meanings as the sole ends of his inquiry, but this does not mean that he would disregard them. Hence, it is difficult to see where there is a contradiction between meaning and causation.

(2) *Meaning in the two noncausal senses cannot in practice remain completely noncausal.* It may be seen that meaning in the two noncausal senses of the term disregards the actuality of the connection between psychic entities. What follows from this is that a concern with meaning only in these senses does not allow for a concern with a search for personal truth in the sense of a wish to discover the real nature of one's psyche. As Schafer (1976, p. 304) explains, when analysts arrive at interpretations of what the patient was "really" doing "we [analysts] are using the word 'really' to indicate that as psychoanalysts, we are satisfied with the type and degree of intelligibility we have achieved through this restatement." But once personal truth is put aside in this way, once the concern shifts to mere intelligibility, why should the patient be concerned with such an understanding of meaning? Why should she, for example, care or acknowledge that there is a connection between one's fear of headaches and one's sense of guilt if this is not *really true*?

Furthermore, if psychoanalysis is not concerned with personal truth; if it is concerned with a literary creation like "pattern-making" as Spence suggests or with some form of elucidation of subjective experience, then this disregard for the real facts may be justified only if patients are so informed. But if this information is not directly conveyed to the patients—and it is my impression that it is not—then patients will continue to believe that what they are dealing with in their understanding of their meanings is truth and hence causal relations between psychic events. People will continue to believe that when they speak of the meanings of their fears and their senses of guilt—that when they say "this means that" and "this is because of that"—that they are speaking of something real. They will not conclude that they are merely describing a subjective experience or a literary tie. In fact, this "real" and causal way of thinking is so entrenched in our everyday thinking that even were the analyst to inform his patients that she is applying meaning in a noncausal sense only, it is questionable whether this would enable the patient to apply it in that way only.[6] Moreover, it would seem that it is because of this entrenchment that analysts do not inform their patient that they are not talking about real psychic events on the causal level. They are too entrenched in it to do so.

It may also be noted that the neglect of this causal sense of meaning severely constricts our understanding of the individual's predicament and experience. If there really is a sense of guilt that is influencing Jane's fear of her headache, then her predicament is not the same as that of someone who only subjectively experiences this to be the case or creatively decides that this is the case. Thus, if psychoanalysis is concerned with the understanding and formulation of subjective experience, it would seem that a comprehensive understanding of this kind would include the causal level. Since subjective experiences bring about, are brought about by, give birth to, are created from, are responsible for the occurrence of, or, in short, cause and are caused, an account of subjective experience is incomplete unless it also includes causal relations. To be interested in subjective experiences is also to be interested in how subjective experiences are brought about (caused) or influence (cause) other experiences and behaviors. In fact, one may understand a concern with causal meaning, (i.e., with "meaning discovered") not as interest in causes per se, not as a move away from experience, but rather as an interest in acknowledging experience in the most comprehensive and most meaningful way.

In sum, if the causal level of meaning is not involved in the psychoanalytic inquiry, the search for personal truth is limited. This search may not be of interest to the analyst, but patients will be concerned with it nevertheless and thus that level of meaning will implicitly be involved. One reason they will be concerned is because to understand one's subjective experience, to have it acknowledged, is, in part, to recognize the truth regarding the causal influences that underlie it.

A Concluding Note on Meaning and Causation. The Choice Is Not between the Hermeneuticists and Grünbaum. For over a decade Adolph Grünbaum has been denouncing the disregard for causation that is found among the psychoanalytical hermeneuticists. His argument regarding the central role of causation always emerges in the context of the issue of therapeutic efficacy. Psychoanalysis is, according to Grünbaum, a causal theory regarding psychopathology, hence, if the theory were true, then causal explanation would be necessary for cure. The major response to Grünbaum is that he is misconstruing the essential nature of psychoanalysis. Psychoanalysis is not (and some would say never was) concerned with singling out specific causes; it is rather a theory of personal meaning and its integration and hence causation is inconsequential. What I am suggesting here goes beyond these two alternatives. Indeed, psychoanalysis is a theory of personal meaning. It is not concerned with singling out causes in order to facilitate adaptive behavior. Grünbaum 's view of psychoanalysis and its aims is limited. And yet the conclusion to be drawn from this is not that we should put aside causation. On the contrary, it is because we are in search of meaning in the most comprehensive sense of the term that it is necessary that we concern ourselves with causation. It is here that the hermeneuticists are misguided. Personal meaning should not, and in a deep sense cannot, be dissociated from causation. If we are after personal meaning, if we honestly desire self-understanding, then we cannot be satisfied with description or creation of meaning. If these are the aims of psychoanalysis, then it must involve a process of discovery of the meanings that are real in us and that are forming and influencing—that is, causing—the nature of our experience.

Conclusion Concerning the Hermeneuticist Critique of Positivism

The present study of the hermeneuticists critique of "positivism" reveals that their rejection of the natural science approach to psychoanalysis is founded on a misguided conceptualization of this approach. In contrast to their claims, the concern with objective facts and causes does not require an extreme constriction of the field of interest to the exclusion of subjectivity and meaning. One may maintain a scientific perspective, be interested in the facts, including the facts of experience, psychic reality, and the causal processes that take place therein, and have as one's utmost aim the elucidation of meaning and the understanding of subjectivity. In fact, it has been argued here that such a scientific perspective is necessary for the attainment of this aim.

The Hermeneuticist Conception

The hermeneuticist approach to psychoanalysis has, in effect, been put forth in this discussion of the "positivistic" approach. The essentials of the psychoanalytic hermeneuticism are presented as the inversion of, and the only alternative to, what its supporters consider to be the scientific approach to psychoanalysis. They are not concerned with facts, they are aware that there are no data that are not molded by theory; they are concerned with meanings rather than with causes, and so on. Of course, individual hermeneuticists have evolved specific and more complex elaborations of these essentials, but it is these essentials that constitute the heart of the approach.[7]

In terms of the different conceptions of meaning that I have pointed to earlier, the hermeneuticist approach can be seen to fall primarily into that of "meaning created." Although some emphasize the experiential descriptive aspect of meaning (Atwood & Stolorow, 1984; Klein, 1976), as a rule what is distinctive of this approach is their focus on the narrative, on the coherent storyline, on pattern-making (Schafer, 1983, Spence, 1982a). What determines meaning here is the thematic tie between mental contents that allows for a coherent story.

The limitations of this view were already discussed. It was seen that its most basic formulations regarding facts, causation, meaning, the possibilities of relating to these in the psychoanalytic setting, and so on, were all of a highly problematic nature. Moreover, it became difficult to see how in practice their limited view of meaning could be maintained or how it could be justified in the light of the aims of psychoanalysis. People seek actual meaning, not created meaning, and will continue to do so even in the face of warnings that that is not really what we are involved in. Psychoanalysis, if regarded as an approach to self-understanding, cannot justifiably attempt to thwart this search. Ultimately, we must assume either that causal conceptions of meaning are indeed implicitly emerging into the hermeneutic psychoanalytic setting or that a rather strange process, one based on a literary view of the person, rather than a real and causal one, is taking place contrary to the one of the patient's basic intentions.

Perhaps one reason the hermeneuticists have introduced this view has to do with the difficulties that have been encountered in justifying the foundations of psychoanalysis according to what they consider acceptable scientific criteria. In the face of their conviction that psychoanalysis is a theory and practice of real value and their feeling that they have failed to prove it conclusively in a scientifically acceptable way, the hermeneuticists have resolved the possible dissonance that may emerge here by affording psychoanalysis a special nonscientific status. That is, when the psychoanalytic propositions failed to meet the criteria of the natural sciences, rather than acknowledge failure of the theory, a psychoanalytical hermeneuticist position developed that claimed that the propositions were not really scientific to begin with, and therefore never had to meet the criteria. Psychoanalysis is to be considered a discipline of intrinsic value whether or not it stands up to the scientific criteria. To maintain this special status, however, the hermeneuticists had to drastically reformulate very basic propositions. Hence their assertions that there is no fact of the matter regarding psychic events, that in psychoanalysis meanings cannot relate to causal processes, and so on.

It may be seen that there are two basic alternatives to this questionable maneuver: (1) to conclude that since psychoanalysis *does* belong to the natural sciences it cannot count as an acceptable theory because of its failure to stand up to scientific criteria; thus the intuitions regarding its value were misguided; and (2) to continue to hold on to these intuitions and strive toward the justification of the theory in accord with scientific standards. One way of doing so is by deepening our understanding of the various possibilities of justification that exist within the bounds of science.

It is my view that this latter alternative must be explored to the fullest before psychoanalysis is deemed an untenable scientific theory, or conversely a theory of irrefutable, and yet questionable, value as a special variety of a hermeneutic discipline. I thus turn now to the exploration of the various possibilities of justification.

The Issue of Justification

Some Basic Forms of Justification and Their Misportrayal in the Hermeneuticist Conception

As stated earlier, the justification of a theory is the means or procedure by which it is supported—that is, the empirical evidence, reasonings, and other considerations through which it is shown to be acceptable. The issue of how a theory is to be justified is far from trivial, since it depends on one's conception of the nature of theories and of evidence, on which views may widely vary. This applies to psychoanalytic theories as well. The issue of how a psychoanalytic theory is to be justified depends on the issue of what exactly a psychoanalytic theory is. As we have seen, the latter issue is highly disputed in the context of the spurious debate between hermeneuticism and "positivism." Thus it is not surprising that the debate over how psychoanalysis is to be justified is currently (mis)portrayed as taking place between a positivistic conception of justification on the one hand, and a hermeneutic conception of justification on the other.

The "positivistic" side in the debate is viewed as based on the model of science, which is focused on the empirical testing of single propositions or statements. According to this view, in order to test a theory one has to examine separately each of the propositions that the theory is comprised of, and justify each of them on the basis of empirical observations, or more specifically, on the basis of theory-free data (Home, 1966; Renik, 1998; Schafer, 1976, 1983).

The other approach to justification, the alternative that the hermeneuticists offer to this simplistic empiricist approach, says that in order to justify a theory one needs to show that the statements that make up the theory are coherent among themselves rather than that they can be based on empirical facts, that what justifies a given proposition is its coherence with a broader set of accepted propositions (Sherwood, 1969; Spence, 1982a; Ricouer, 1981).

Ricouer (1981, p. 271) contends that what this means is that "a good psychoanalytic explanation must be coherent with the theory, or if one prefers, it must conform to Freud's psychoanalytic system." Other hermeneuticists have emphasized, however, that the theory (or explanation) should not only be coherent but should also explain all relevant data and not be contradicted by them (see Strenger, 1991, p. 187). This latter emphasis, however, is somewhat strange. It suggests that the empirical data have a special status. A statement regarding observational data is not considered here to be just another proposition (one about observations) that is to be accepted or rejected depending on whether it coheres with the theoretical propositions. Rather, the theoretical propositions must account for the data. This emphasis is strange since (as we have seen) the hermeneuticists question the very availability of hard data and consider there to be no matter of fact regarding them.

I will now demonstrate how just as the choice between "meaning" and "causation" that was put forth by the hermeneuticists is misleading, so this dichotomy of forms of justification is overly simplistic and at points misleading as well. In particular, by regarding "positivism" as the representative of the scientific method, hermeneuticists misrepresent the wealth of possibilities that exist within the framework of science. I will not present here an exposition of the range of theories of justification that have evolved over the years. I will instead briefly present some very basic forms of justification that exist in the domain of science.

To this end let us first put the most basic distinction regarding justification into more appropriate terms. The hermeneuticist strategy for justification through coherence alone is commonly called *the Coherence theory of justification*. It predates hermeneuticism, and contains several alternative versions. Coherence theory of justification may be more appropriately contrasted not with a positivistic form of justification, but rather with the much broader approach of so-called *Foundationalism*. Both approaches contain a variety of subtheories, but for our purpose it would be sufficient to divide Foundationalism into two: Atomistic and Holistic Foundationalist theories of justification. Thus, in the present discussion, we will focus on four theories of justification: Coherentism versus Foundationalism, the latter of which is divided into Atomistic and Holistic forms. "Positivism" is associated with the Atomistic brand of Foundationalism, and does not by any means exhaust the range of alternatives to the hermeneutic form of justification. As I now clarify these distinctions, I will focus on two interrelated dimensions: the status of the data and the criteria of justification (see Figure 1.2).[8]

Foundationalist Theories of Justification

Foundationalism is the view that theories are justified when they are properly based on a foundation that has a high degree of certainty—according to some versions, that is even infallible. The idea is that if a foundation is certain, then any theory that is properly based on it will be certain too. Perhaps the analogy of a house is fruitful here. Just as a house must be based on a stable foundation in order not to crumble, theories too need to be based on a solid foundation in order not to crumble, that is, in order to be justified. Hence the term "Foundationalism."

Figure 1.2. Justification Distinctions Chart

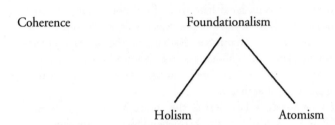

What is the nature of the foundation on which a theory can be built? So-called Rationalist theories require a foundation made of first principles derived from reason alone. By pure reason, without the aid of any empirical observation, one is supposed to discover the foundation of our knowledge. An alternative approach, or rather cluster of approaches, generically called Empiricism, holds that theories about the world should rest on empirical observations. By looking at the world, whether with the naked eye or with the aid of scientific instruments and methods, we can discover basic data about the phenomena in question. On the basis of these data—which is to say, propositions describing the findings made through observations—we can construct theories.[9] A theory is justified when it is properly based upon a foundation of empirical data. Since psychoanalysis is a field that relies on observations (clinical ones), I will not further mention the Rationalist version of Foundationalism. And for the sake of simplicity, when I henceforth speak of Foundationalism I will mean only Empiricist Foundationalism, that is, Foundationalism according to which justified theories are based on the foundation of empirical data.

According to Foundationalism in this qualified (Empiricist) sense, observational data are not like any other proposition or belief. On the contrary, the observational data are the foundations for our knowledge about the world, whereas theoretical propositions compose the superstructure built on these foundations. We investigators find through observations various data, and our theoretical propositions are justified when they account for the data. Various Foundationalist approaches differ on the degree to which they consider the data to be theory-free and infallible. The specifics of these subdivisions do not concern us here, but it should be recognized that it is commonly accepted among almost all modern-day Foundationalists that theory does influence the data.

Nevertheless, they hold that the data has a special status such that it could serve as a foundation for the theoretical propositions.

Here we may turn to the distinction between two versions of Foundationalism: Atomism and Holism. *Atomistic (Foundationalist)* approaches to justification hold that a proposition of a theory is justified if it can be based on, and explain the observational data in some specified way.[10] What is atomistic here is that one attempts to justify each theoretical proposition in isolation from any other. The justification for acceptance of Freud's second theory of anxiety, for example, will be assessed in isolation from any of his other propositions. Similarly, the justification of a specific interpretation of a dream can be determined without reference to any broader framework. Logical positivism, which was popular in the first half of the century, held this foundational-atomistic theory of justification, and it is with it that the hermeneuticists seem to be taking issue. For the past fifty years, however, there are few, even among the most rigorous scientists, who would admittedly subscribe to such a view.

In contrast to this Atomistic version of Foundationalism, there is the *Holistic (Foundationalist)* approach to justification. Like the Atomistic version, this approach too holds that theories are justified when they are shown to account for the observational data. However, according to the Holistic approach, it is never individual isolated propositions that are justified, but rather larger chunks of theories, or even entire theories. This is because what explain observational data are never single individual theoretical propositions, but rather entire theories. It is the theory as a whole that needs to be shown to account for the observational data as a whole, and hence to be justified. Single propositions would then be justified if they cohere with the broader theoretical body and their addition to it enhances the capacity of the broader theory to account for the data.

There are various considerations supporting this Holistic approach to justification. According to one type of consideration, specific propositions assume their meaning only within the framework of a broader theory (Quine, 1960). Since single propositions isolated from their context have no meaning, it is impossible to justify them in isolation from the theory in which they are embedded. Another line of thought suggests that any proposition in a theory can "hook up" to the data only with the help of other statements. Thus, even a straightforward proposition about observable states of affairs requires reliance on theories regarding the methods and tools by way of which the observations are being made. Hence, many propositions in the theory, if not all of them, rely on each other in their relationship to the observational, empirical foundation on which they are supposed to be based. Accordingly, any single proposition taken in isolation may not have sufficient grounds for its justification; available considerations may not conclusively show that the acceptance of the proposition is warranted. And yet, according to this approach, the proposition may nevertheless be justified. Its justification would rest on the relationship of the proposition to the network of propositions in which it resides: It is justified because it coheres with other (or even all other) propositions in the theory and, when taken together with this broader body of propositions, is properly based on (and hence justified by) the data. In the context of psychoanalysis, adherence to this form of justification would, for example, lead to questions regarding how well Freud's second theory of anxiety, or how well a specific interpretation regarding anxiety, fits with the broader network of propositions (in the general theory or regarding the specific person) and how well this whole network accounts for the available data.

Coherence Theories of Justification

In contrast to the Foundationalist theories of justification there are Coherence theories of justification. These theories emphasize that the commonsensical (traditional and no longer acceptable) idea that we human investigators have access to raw, pre-theoretical data cannot be maintained. There are no such things as pure, theory-free observations in which the observer merely reads off raw data from the facts. They stress that since we always observe the world from the perspective of a specific way of understanding, a specific conceptual scheme, whatever we observe is already shaped by our theories. We are locked, so to speak, within our theories and conceptual schemes, and our observations, are in fact, observational propositions (propositions about observations), which, like all other propositions, are couched within a specific theory.

Since proponents of Coherence theories of justification emphasize the great influence of our theories on observations, they draw the conclusion that propositions about the empirical data should not be considered to have a status different from that of any other propositions within a theory. Propositions about data are regarded as theory-laden, and hence part of the theory in question. It is not as if there is empirical data that could serve as the foundation for theoretical propositions. Rather, propositions about the data are considered to be like any other proposition. If all propositions are theory-laden, then in order to justify a theoretical proposition one cannot base it on the fact that it accounts for the data, for these too are not theory-free. Is there any way of supporting a theoretical proposition if everything available to us is necessarily part of a theory? The answer that Coherence theory offers is that all propositions are justified according to the nature of their relationships to the other propositions. Namely, a proposition is justified if adding it to one's theory (i.e., to one's set of theoretical propositions) will make the theory more coherent. To give a psychoanalytical example, if Freud's second theory of anxiety, whereby anxiety is to be considered a signal—rather than a transformation of libido, as Freud believed regarding his first theory—enhances the coherence of the overall theory, then the belief in this new addition is justified. In this context, "the evidence" that Freud procures in favor of the addition is just another proposition, an observational one, one that like any other part of the theory may have to be thrown out if it does not preserve the coherence of the theory (Dancy, 1985, p. 118). Thus, if propositions about observations of anxiety states do not cohere with the theory, we may interpret these observations as mistaken. We may reinterpret certain observations of anxiety to be only seemingly expressions of anxiety if the observation of them as such does not cohere with the theory of anxiety being proposed. Of course, this theory of justification would require (for the sake of coherence) that an explanation be provided of why what was not really anxiety appeared to be so.

The Relationship between the Holistic Foundationalist Approach and the Coherence Theory of Justification

We noted earlier that hermeneuticists emphasize the role of coherence in their approach to justification. But in this unitary focus what is blurred is an important distinction that is to be found between the Holistic Foundationalist approach to justification and the Coherence theory of justification. Both hold that individual propositions cannot be evaluated for their justification unless they are seen as part of the broader framework of the theory. In other words, both would agree that only entire theories (or parts of theories), not individual propositions, could be justified. Furthermore, both can be understood as requiring coherence in order to justify the acceptance of propositions. Doesn't this mean that they are virtually indistinguishable?

The answer is that there is a fundamental difference between the two, one that, unfortunately, has been (for the most part) neglected in the review of Freud's approach to justification. The difference lies in the role of empirical data in the two approaches. As previously explained, the Holistic approach is a version of foundationalism, which demands that a theory be based on empirical data in order to be justified. The data, therefore, have a special status: They constitute the foundation on which the theory should rest. Coherentist theories, on the other hand, do not consider the data to hold any special status. Data descriptions, being presumably theory-laden, are nothing but another part of the theory equivalent to any other part, rather than being the foundation of the theory. After all, according to the Coherentist approach, theories have no epistemological foundation. A theory supports itself, so to speak, through internal coherence, rather than being based on a foundation. This means that data propositions are judged like any other part of the theory: They must cohere with the rest of the theory and, if they fail to do so, they should be rejected or modified to enhance the overall coherence of the theory.

This difference in the status of the data is a sharp one. The Holistic investigator may modify the theoretical propositions in order to account for the data—or, if you wish, she can modify the theory to make it coherent with the data—but not the other way around. She cannot modify the data to fit the theory. To be sure, the data need not be completely immune from error. A Holistic researcher may sometimes discard a piece of data, as, say, a measurement error, on the ground that it is too unlikely—being too incoherent with the rest of the observational and theoretical propositions. But rejection of data may only be done in special cases, and cannot be done systematically in order to fit the theory, as the Coherence theory implies. In this sense, in the Holistic approach there is asymmetry between data propositions and theoretical propositions: the latter rely on the former, and not the other way around; the latter can be modified to account for (or cohere with) the former, but not vice versa. Unlike in Coherence theories, here coherence is not sought as an ultimate aim in its own right. It is not the coherence in itself that is the source of justification, but rather it serves as a means for accounting for a privileged class of propositions, namely those describing the data. There are facts that are considered to serve as the foundation, and it is the task of the theoretical propositions to explain them. When they do so, only then are we justified in accepting the proposition.

All this implies that although both approaches use coherence as a criterion for justifying a theory, this criterion nevertheless plays a different role in each of the two. In the Coherence theory of justification, coherence is the only criterion for evaluating the acceptability of a theory. In contrast, in Holistic Foundationalism, coherence is only one of two criteria for evaluating a theory. For, in addition to the issue of coherence, theories are also evaluated in accordance with how well they account for the data. Hence, the Coherence theory is—as its name implies—indeed a theory of coherence; justification is nothing more than demonstration of coherence. Holistic Foundationalism, on the other hand, is a theory that *uses* the criterion of coherence, but only as one element in a broader conception of the nature of justification.

Once the relationship between these different theories is clarified it may be seen that the very fact that the hermeneuticists emphasize coherence does not in itself require that they be classified as Coherentists. They could be considered so only to the extent that they do not regard accountability for the observational data to be an essential criterion for justification. As we noted earlier, it is precisely on this point that the hermeneuticists seem to be unclear. They emphasize the theory-ladenness of all psychoanalytic observations, and at best consider the facts to be interpretations. But at the same time they seem to suggest (some very explicitly) that the justification of our more theoretical propositions should in part be determined by their capacity to explain the facts.

One further comment on the criterion of coherence is in place here. When one speaks of making a proposition coherent with a larger body of propositions, the question naturally arises: How large a body? The answer is that one can make a proposition coherent with various sizes of contexts: with a small group of propositions about the anxiety of a given patient, with a theory of anxiety, with the entire theory of psychoanalysis, or even with our overall conception of the world. We may say, therefore, that the criterion of coherence can be used (both in Holistic Foundationalism and in Coherentist theories) more locally or atomistically, or alternatively more holistically. This also means that the difference between Atomistic and Holistic Foundationalism is more a matter of degree than a matter of dichotomy.

Truth and Justification

So far we dealt with the issue of justification: What is it that justifies an investigator in maintaining a given proposition or theory? But note that we have not yet dealt directly or systematically with the issue of *truth*, an issue that is closely tied to the issue of justification and very relevant to the question of whether psychoanalytic exploration does or should take place within the framework of natural science. Ordinarily, we are interested in theories that are justified only because we wish to approach the truth as much as possible. Presumably, if we are careful to opt for theories that are properly justified, we are more likely to approach the truth. This raises the question: What is truth? What does it mean to say of a theory that it is true? Naturally, there are several different views on the nature of truth.

We may begin to explore these views by recognizing the relationship between the different approaches to justification and the issue of truth. Foundationalism, whether Holistic or Atomistic, in its attempt to separate data from theory and to make the latter approximate the former, implies that a theory is true when it corresponds to the facts. This is the *Correspondence* theory of truth. According to this picture, there are facts on the one hand and theory on the other, and the theory is true when it mirrors the facts. It is because of this conception of truth that theories are said to be justified when they cohere with, or account for, the observational data, which are presumably samples of the facts. Our observations tell us about objects out there in the world, and our theories are systematic accounts of these observations. That is, there is a correspondence between our theoretical propositions and reality (external or internal). According to an Atomistic approach to justification, this correspondence can be tested for each theoretical proposition by itself by applying the appropriate method (e.g., a deductive method). According to a Holistic approach to justification the entire theory would have to be shown to account for the entire body of observations. Either way, the basic idea is that theories are designed to correspond to the phenomenon under investigation.

Just as Foundationalist theories of justification naturally go together with the Correspondence theory of truth, the Coherence theory of justification naturally goes hand in hand with another conception of the nature of truth, namely, the *Coherence* theory of truth—not to be confused with the Coherentist theory of *justification*. Indeed, various thinkers have suggested that the adoption of a Coherentist theory of justification requires the adoption of a Coherentist theory of truth (Dancy, 1985). Regarding the Coherence theory of truth, the idea is that in order for a theory to be true it need not correspond to anything outside itself. Rather, it has to maximally cohere within itself. This theory of truth goes well together with the Coherence theory of justification because if a true theory is one that is maximally coherent, then naturally in order to justify a theory we need to show that it is internally coherent. And, vice versa, the denial of a special foundational status to observational data makes it more difficult to hold a Correspondence theory of truth. It does not, however, make it an impossibility. Several leading philosophers in this area have argued that a Coherentist theory of justification could be accompanied by a Correspondence theory of truth (Ewing, 1934; Lehrer, 1974; Rescher, 1973). This position would mean that the sole criterion of coherence helps us in achieving correspondence with the facts (i.e., truth according to the Correspondence theory of truth). Our theories are more likely to correspond to the facts if they are justified in the Coherentist manner, that is, if the theoretical and observational propositions of which they are composed are made maximally coherent.

All this points to the fact that concern with coherence, either within a Foundationalist or Coherentist model, does not do away with the notion of truth. But as we saw earlier in our discussion of meaning, it would seem that the psychoanalytical hermeneuticists do in fact do away with the notion of truth. There appears to be some confusion and disagreement among hermeneuticists on this point (see Hanly, 1990; Wallerstein, 1986, pp. 422–423,), but there is one clear line of thought that suggests that a search for coherence must take the place of a search for truth. This is expressed most clearly in Schafer's comment (1976, p. 204) mentioned earlier that "the word 'really' . . . indicate[s] that . . . we are satisfied with the degree of intelligibility we have achieved." What is stated here is that "really" is a tag that we give when we have attained intelligibility and what is not considered here is that intelligibility may indicate that we have arrived at something real. Psychoanalytical hermeneuticists, who claim that psychoanalytic theories are not concerned with truth, should therefore not be seen as Coherentists concerning truth. They may be Coherentists about justification (i.e., they may hold that a justified theory is a coherent theory), but they are anti-realist about truth (i.e., they hold that the truth of a theory is something that does not exist or at least cannot be achieved).

Meaning, Truth, Justification, and the Hermeneuticist Position

These very basic and broad distinctions between different forms of justification and of truth are important because they dispel the simplistic division of the theoretical field within psychoanalysis into two—a positivistic approach and an approach based solely on coherence. What could be classified as scientific theories of justification extends over quite a broad range. Although the Atomistic approach does come close to that of logical positivism, the Holistic approach, in its focus on a network of propositions and the value of the coherence between them, is far from it.

The dichotomy is further dispelled as we recognize that coherence may be used in different ways. Concern with coherence does not necessarily imply the rejection of a scientific framework of investigation, as the hermeneuticists sometimes claim. First, one can use the criterion of coherence as part of a Holistic Foundationalist program, which seeks to create a theory that corresponds to the facts. (To be sure, it seems at times that the hermeneuticists do in fact adopt such a Foundationalist approach, an approach commonly accepted in the natural sciences.) Second, even if one rejects Foundationalism and adopts coherence as a criteria for accepting theories—for example, for *justification*—one may still hold a Correspondence theory of—*truth*. In this case, coherence may be considered an indication of, or a step toward, correspondence with objective reality (internal or external).[11] Lastly, even if one accepts a Coherentist approach to truth (i.e., that a theory that is true is one that is maximally coherent), this still does not amount to rejecting the notion of truth. For it may still mean that there is some ideal overall theory of our world that is maximally coherent, and that by scientific means we can approach it more and more. All these three uses of coherence are consistent with the scientific enterprise.

Alternately, coherence can be applied in a way that reflects a rejection of a scientific view. When there is no longer a concern with truth, when coherence is sought for its own sake, when we accept propositions because they cohere but without any view to the deeper understanding of actual reality, then it may be difficult to speak of a scientific perspective.

All this sheds light on the position of psychoanalytic hermeneuticists. Hermeneuticists have claimed that the role of the psychoanalyst is to create a *coherent* story, not a *true* story, of psychic reality. As we have just seen, the two notions in no way contradict each other, as the hermeneuticists seem to think. One can be concerned with building a coherent picture of the patient's life, and at the same time aim for discovering the truth. On the contrary, as we have seen, it is very reasonable to regard coherence as a crucial criterion that points in the direction of truth. Indeed, this is precisely what scientists do when they create their theories.

This means that when the psychoanalyst attempts to create a coherent story of a patient, or of patients in general, he or she can be portrayed as seeking the truth about the psychic reality of the patient. The analyst's descriptions of the patient's unconscious, anxieties, hidden meanings, and so on, need not be seen as useful fictions, but rather as genuine attempts to formulate a true description of the facts about the patient's psyche. That the analyst is aiming for coherence does not in any way mean that he or she is not aiming for truth.

The hermeneuticist may reply with other arguments attempting to show that it makes no sense to speak about the truth regarding psychic facts. Earlier we already saw some of these arguments: Psychic states are subjective, or unobservable, or theory-laden and therefore are not matters of fact. As we have seen, these arguments are fallacious when applied specifically to psychoanalytic theory. There seems to be nothing unreasonable in attempting to discover the facts about psychic reality—as subjective, unobservable, and theory-laden as they might be. The fact that psychic events are subjective hardly implies that there is no fact of the matter about them. It only means that they are in some sense within the subject. The fact that subjective states are not directly observable also does not imply that the facts about them cannot be investigated. The investigation of realities that are not directly observable is precisely the domain of science. Just as the physicist investigates quarks and black holes that cannot be directly observed, and just as the biologist investigates the behavior or organic molecules that cannot be directly observed, the psychoanalyst investigates psychic facts that are not directly observable. Lastly, the fact that observations of psychic realities are always done from the perspective of some theory does not mean that these realities cannot be investigated. If the idea is that we are doomed to remain within our human conceptual scheme and can never extract ourselves to the real ultimate Truth, the answer is that this should apply to physics, chemistry, biology, and all other sciences. The fact that science is possible shows that theory-ladenness is not an obstacle to science. It simply implies that what science investigates is the-world-as-portrayed-by-a-human-conceptual-scheme. A simple look around us may discover that that world is obviously not devoid of hard facts. That the door over there is open, that hydrogen has one electron, that Jane is anxious, and that Joe is suffering from the effect of a childhood trauma—these may very well be facts only within the human world, the world of our conceptual scheme or our theories. But whether or not they are so, it nevertheless is the case that within our world they are hard facts that can be investigated responsibly by scientific and other means, theorized about, and explained. Within the world we humans share, our intersubjective world—whether it is the ultimate truth or a result of human ways of looking—there are hard facts.

These arguments are not meant to be a conclusive proof against hermeneuticism. The point is rather that, upon careful analysis of basic notions, the hermeneuticist's professed wariness of truth and facts seems to be premature. *Before despairing of the psychoanalytic attempt to uncover psychic reality, we should first examine closely and see whether psychoanalytic theories can be justified for their truth. This is indeed the purpose of the present work.* As I will show, the attempt to understand psychic facts is far from hopeless.

We have seen how the hermeneuticist position with respect to truth is intimately tied to the hermeneuticist notion of meaning. If hermeneuticists reject the possibility of uncovering the truth about patients' psychic reality, it follows that they are not trying to *discover* psychic meanings in the patient's psyche. All they can do is weave or create meanings, or alternatively point to the patient's experience of something meaning this or that, since the truth about meanings, about the actual connections between psychic entities that exist in the mind, is allegedly inaccessible to us. In the terminology coined earlier, hermeneuticists can talk about what I called "meaning created" or "meaning experienced," but not about "meaning discovered." This is indeed what hermeneuticists claim to be doing. However, if as I argued, psychoanalysts are justified in their claim to discover facts about patients' psyche, then what they can do is discover actual meaning-connections that reside in patients' psyche. In other words, it is then legitimate to ask questions about the causal connections—what brought about what—in the patient. The examination of the psychoanalytic theory regarding the meaning of the dream, which will be carried out in the present study, will focus precisely on this causal, discovered, kind of meaning.

Two steps, however, remain ahead of us before proceeding with this examination. We must first briefly delineate where Freud stands in relation to the issues of meaning and of truth. In this context I will in passing make a general statement regarding the nature of Freud's project of justification. In these remarks my intention will not be to substantiate my understanding of Freud on these broad issues—this would take us too far afield—but rather to prepare the reader for the kinds of "meaning" and "truth" that we will be dealing with in our indepth exploration of Freud's attempt to justify his theory in the coming chapter. In the course of that chapter the nature of Freud's use of these terms will become more apparent and will be further discussed. Second, we must examine the studies that have already explored the question of whether Freud's dream theory has been adequately justified. This will make it apparent that there is room for further exploration of this area.

PART II: A BRIEF OUTLINE OF FREUD'S STANCE ON "MEANING," "TRUTH," AND "JUSTIFICATION"

Many writers make passing reference to Freud's views on meaning, but there have been few attempts to classify his use of the term relative to other possible uses.[12] Now that we have seen the range of different meanings ascribed to the term meaning within psychoanalysis, the task of clarifying Freud's position is made much more simple.

Freud, of course, relied on the use of the term "meaning" in a great variety of ways. In order to carry on any form of discourse, for example, he must be concerned with meaning in semantic and pragmatic senses of the term. In carrying on debates with his colleagues regarding the meaning of certain concepts, his concern with meaning may have also remained on the level of various forms of relationships between contents. But these kinds of meanings were not part of Freud's focal interest. His focal interest, the kind of meaning that he struggled to discern or discover, was meaning in terms of the relationship between psychic events. This interest was maintained both on the level of theory and on the level of the individual meanings that Freud sought to understand in his work with his patients as well as in his self-analysis.

Our earlier distinction between the "meaning of the statement" and the "meaning of stating" should be recalled here. Although this point has not been emphasized in the literature, Freud's interest in meaning as the relationship between psychic entities refers to both these kinds of meanings. That is, when speaking of meaning he referred to both the nature of relationships between psychic entities that were being expressed in the statement itself, and the nature of the relationships between such entities that were expressed in the factor that caused the stating of the statement. For example, when Freud dreams that "R. was my uncle" (Freud, 1900, p. 138) he first wonders as to "What could that mean?" On the basis of a variety of considerations, none of which having anything to do with motivations, he concludes that "there could be no doubt that I really did mean that my friend R. was a simpleton—like my Uncle Josef" (p. 139). This is the meaning of the statement. It is the unconscious intention that is finding expression in the statement. Later Freud addresses the issue of what motivated the expression of this meaning. Here another meaning comes to fore—Freud's wish to receive the title of professor. The motivational tie (i.e., the wish), which is the meaning of stating, is considered by Freud to be a prominent sense of meaning, not only in the dream, but in all contexts in which motives are involved and meanings are to be discerned. At this point it may be seen how the "meaning of stating" and the "meaning of the statement" refer to two levels within the causal network. The motive (e.g., the wish to be a professor) causes a range of ideas (e.g., R. is a simpleton) to cause the appearance of the manifest thought (e.g., R. was my uncle). Hence the meaning of the manifest thought can be considered in terms of both.[13]

For Freud meaning was not something to simply be read off experience, nor was it something to be created. Undoubtedly Freud was concerned with meaning *discovered*. When Freud wrote to his friend and colleague Fliess, "Do you suppose that some day one will read on a marble tablet on this house: Here on July 24, 1895, the secret of the dream revealed itself to Dr. Sigm. Freud" (Freud, 1985, p. 417), he was telling him of the revelation of the real connections between psychic entities that underlie the dream. If Freud's finding was merely that of the possibility of experiencing meanings in relation to the dream or of weaving together various themes to form a coherent meaning, it would be difficult to consider this a revelation. The existence of these possibilities is self-evident. What is not self-evident and what Freud considered to be his revelation was that he could discover the actual connections in the mind that were responsible for the appearance of the dream—the actual connections that motivated its appearance and that were finding expression through it. This focus on the discovery of meaning was of course not limited to the dream. In his attempt to understand the psyche of both the neurotic and the normal individual Freud's concern was always with the discovery of the actual connections that exist within the mind.

This focus on the discovery of actual meanings is intimately tied to Freud's concern with truth. Freud was trying to discover the truth about psychic reality. In this sense Freud was a realist with respect to psychic states. In other words, he believed that psychic states, including unconscious, not directly observable ones, and the causal connections between them (i.e., meanings) have independent existence. They are the way they are independently of whether or how we conceive of them. Descriptions and theories about psychic states are true or false depending on facts of the matter. Freud here adopts a Correspondence theory of truth: A theory or a proposition is true if it corresponds to the facts. This position of Freud stands in sharp contrast to the anti-realist positions that we encountered in our discussion of psychoanalytical hermeneuticism, according to which there is no fact of the matter concerning psychic states. Furthermore, it also stands in contrast to those adhering to the Coherence theory of truth, according to which all that is required of a theory for it to be true is that it be internally coherent, and not that it correspond to extra-theoretical facts. To be sure, Freud, as we will soon see, sometimes uses coherence as a criterion for the acceptability (justification) of a theory, but his aim is to have the theory correspond to the facts. This might be taken to imply that Freud employs a Coherence theory of justification, but, as will become apparent in the next chapter, Freud remained loyal to a Foundationalist program, which, as we have seen, can also employ the coherence criterion within its Holistic version.

Were the current study written some twenty years ago there would have been no reason to make this point. It would have been obvious that this is Freud's position. Today, however, with the growing popularity of new perspectives on meaning, especially that of the psychoanalytical hermeneuticists, it has became necessary to reemphasize this basic position of Freud. In light of these new perspectives as well as the reinterpretations of Freud in the light of them it has become necessary to make clear that Freud's concern is indeed with the discovery of actual meaning. Here the contrast is both with the notion (a mistaken one) that Freud was actually concerned with the other forms of meaning, such as "meaning created" (e.g., Ricouer, 1971), and with the notion (equally mistaken) that Freud was not concerned with meaning at all; that his concern was *instead* with causes, or blind forces, biological frameworks, and other non-meaning related entities (Klein, 1976). It has become necessary to shatter the so-called "positivistic" confines into which Freud has been placed in recent years and to state in no unclear terms that meaning and cause do not contradict each other, that one does not come at the expense of the other, and that Freud's search for causes, his elaboration of the real underlying causal network, was and is part and parcel of the deep and complex theory of meaning that he was evolving. It has become necessary to reassert that Freud's concern is with truth, with developing propositions and theories that correspond to the facts, and that this is a legitimate and even worthy endeavor for psychoanalysis.

The question that we now face is whether Freud's assertion that he has discovered the secret of the dream is justified. More specifically, the question is whether the meanings of dreams that Freud arrives at are indeed meanings according to Freud's use of the term. Can we know this to be the case? In the following chapters I will explore this question, beginning with Freud's own attempts to justify his theory. There we will encounter the different forms of Foundationalism to which Freud adhered and explore the degree to which Freud in these approaches succeeded to justify his dream theory. This will lead to the exploration of alternate paths and to a new understanding of the epistemological foundations of the psychoanalytic theory of dreams.

Before turning to my exploration let us first look at the two available significant studies that have already explored this issue. This will clarify the place of the current study.

PART III: CRITICAL STUDIES OF THE EPISTEMOLOGY OF FREUD'S THEORY OF DREAM INTERPRETATION

In the psychoanalytic literature the examination of Freud's theories, the understanding of their foundations, has usually taken one of two forms—descriptive or dynamic.[14] In the present context of the foundations of the theory of dreams the descriptive form of understanding is found primarily in the numerous papers, as well as several manuscripts, that have articulated the basic *structure* of Freud's ideas on dreams and their later evolutions (Altman, 1969; Edelson, 1972; Grinstein, 1983; Nagera et al., 1969; Sloane, 1979). These have explicated and clarified Freud's ideas on wish-fulfillment, the nature of the various forms of dream work, the psychological model that underlies it, and so on. The descriptive form of understanding is also found in attempts to explain or clarify the *place* of the dream theory within the broader theoretical edifice as well as in attempts to elaborate the *clinical* basis of Freud's ideas on dreams (Gay, 1988; Jones, 1953).

The other form of understanding, the dynamic form, focuses on the personal meaning of the dream theory to Freud. Here stress is laid on what the theory means in terms of its satisfying various needs of Freud's. That is, to understand the foundations of the theory is to dynamically understand Freud's ambitions (Welsh, 1994), his need to mourn his father (Kris, 1954; Schur, 1972), his need to penetrate the maternal object (Pontalis, 1981), his wish to regain "the desired body of the unpossesed mother" (Anzieu, 1986, p. 155), and so on.

These two forms of understanding, common in the study of the foundations of psychoanalytic thinking within the psychoanalytic literature, are to be contrasted with a third kind of understanding. This is the understanding that is derived from the critical analysis of the theory and of the evidence and arguments brought in its support. Instead of the broader comprehension of statements whose value are taken for granted, which is offered by the first two kinds of understanding, this understanding examines the value of the theory. It is this kind of understanding that allows us to go beyond the clarification of what was intended and why, in order to address the most elementary question of whether the theoretical propositions that are being made are justified and true.

Surprisingly perhaps, this kind of analysis and understanding is scarce in the psychoanalytic literature in relation to the theory of dreams. This may be seen in the fact that the most comprehensive attempt to justify the psychoanalytic theory of dreams, the attempt that has set the foundations of this theory—Freud's (1900) *The Interpretation of Dreams*—has not been subject to intensive critical study. Welsh (1994) in his literary exploration of the book writes:

> The dream book has many times been combed for its autobiographical insights, for its story of the discovery of psychoanalysis, and for its dreams—most of which have been subjected to enthusiastic reinterpretations by other persons. Yet I know of no concerted attempt to examine the book critically so as to take into account . . . the construction of the argument (p. ix).[15]

Although the absence of an in-depth and detailed critical analysis of the psychoanalytic theory of dreams—which may perhaps be understood in the light of a more general absence of such critical study of many fundamental aspects of psychoanalysis—is striking, there are available some more local examinations of Freud's ideas on dreams that indeed touch on the question of whether his ideas in this context are justified. The two most significant works in this are those of Spence (1981) and of Grünbaum (1984, 1993).

Spence's Critique

Spence's questioning of the epistemological foundations of Freud's dream theory reflects the questions of several other theoreticians who have raised objec-

tions in less systematic or directed form.[16] He presents his ideas in a paper entitled "Toward a theory of dream interpretation" (1981). Spence considers
Freud's dream theory to be composed of the basic proposition that the application of the psychoanalytic method to the dream will result in the discovery of
the dream's meanings. The gist of his critique is as follows: Freud's dream
theory is based on ad hoc reasoning. This is revealed by (1) the absence of
"reversibility." That is, it is not likely that an outside judge could reconstruct
the dream on the basis of the latent content that is revealed; (2) a great amount
of detail goes into the formation of the dream's interpretation, rather than a
reduced set of general principles, and this reliance on detail may hide the
absence of general laws governing the process; and (3) sufficient detail will
always make for a convincing interpretation.

Spence seems to see the source of the problem in what he refers to as the
"Correspondence Postulate." According to Spence, this postulate is at the basis
of Freud's method of dream interpretation. It states that

> the associations generated by the dream, in the course of the analytic hour,
> correspond to the dream thoughts which created the dream in the first
> place. The analytic patient, associating in a regressed state of consciousness,
> is presumed to have privileged access to the thoughts and feelings which
> were active at the time when the dream was created. The regression result-
> ing from the specific conditions of the treatment situation is assumed to
> duplicate the regression brought on by sleep, which was, Freud assumed,
> one of the essential features of dream construction. (Spence, 1981, p. 387)

Spence goes on to argue that there is no real basis for this assumption. There is
no way of knowing whether all the associations triggered by the dream are those
that inspired it. Thus, if we rely on these associations, we can never know
whether we have arrived at a true understanding of the dream. We may only
have an illusion of this:

> The question of truth value never arises, however, because familiarity tends
> to be confused with causation. . . . Associations, whether relevant or not,
> have the power to naturalize the dream and link it with known pieces of
> the dreamer's past, present, and future. But we should realize that natural-
> ization does not coincide with explanation; the dream may seem less for-
> eign or exotic or bizarre, but the linking associations have not necessarily
> increased our understanding of why this particular set of images came into
> being at just that moment. . . . A rich yield of associations, whether or not
> they are relevant to the dream, tends to give a sense of successfully decod-
> ing the dream, whereas few associations lead to a sense of failure. (Spence,
> 1981, pp. 387–388)

Spence proceeds to present a form of dream interpretation that would overcome these limitations. The model he suggests is bereft with difficulties, and

since it does not contribute to the understanding of his critique will not be discussed here.

To clarify Spence's critique we may divide his questioning of Freud's dream theory into two: (1) Does Freud's method of dream interpretations satisfy the criteria necessary for justification? Here Spence puts forward his view that justification cannot rely on conviction regarding the interpretations and can be ascertained only if reversibility and general rules of transformation can be discerned. It is not clear that either of these criteria is met. (2) Can Freud's method of dream interpretation provide access to the relevant causal associations (and hence to the meaning of the dream)? Here Spence points to the absence in Freud's writings of criteria that could distinguish between associations that have causal relevance for the dream and those that are mere reactions to it, and the impossibility of knowing whether we have arrived at the true (causal) meaning in the absence of such criteria. We may now turn to the examination of the limitations of Spence's critique.

Spence's view of the criteria that would allow for the justification of Freud's method of interpretation seems unwarrantedly constricted. While clearly, no one, including Freud himself, would consider conviction to be the sole criteria for its justification, the alternative that Spence offers—that for an interpretation to be considered justified it must be possible to reverse the causally relevant latent associations into the dream by means of general rules of association—is rather strange. Such a simplistic hypothetico-deductive approach to explanation is out of place here. If one does not rely on the view that latent thoughts undergo direct transformation in some extremely isolated form (i.e., that each thought has one corresponding image into which it can be transformed), if room is left for the influence of Gestalts, and for multiple forms of expression to any given latent thought, then Spence's criteria for justification cannot be considered relevant. (Spence himself seems to have come to recognize this in a later remark on this issue [Spence, 1982a].) We may have access to the thoughts of an artist that were causally relevant to the painting of a painting, but this does not necessarily mean that we can transform these into the specific painting that the artist painted by applying certain rules of transformation.

Furthermore, Spence does not *show* that such rules of transformation do not exist; he just suggests that this appears to be the case, and that if the rules do exist, they are hidden by much detail. But let us assume that the rules have not been specified. Much of human discourse operates on unspecified rules. In fact, it has been suggested that in the human sciences the prediction of behavior and the understanding of meaning is not based on the application of a specific series of rules, but rather on introspection regarding how I would act or what I would mean were I in the same situation. There is an internal playing out of scenes that provides information about another person (Blackburn, 1984; Gordon, 1987). In any case, it does not seem that Freud's method of dream interpretation suffers from a greater shortage of rules than his method regarding psycho-analysis in general. On the contrary, it would seem that there are more rules in the case of the dream. Hence, were the absence of rules grounds for disqualifica-tion, then Spence would have to disqualify the more general theory of psycho-analysis—and he does not.

Spence's second objection to Freud's dream theory, the objection regard-ing the impossibility of knowing whether in the course of interpretation we are obtaining associations that are indeed causally relevant to the dream, is legiti-mate and serious. However, Spence constricts the problem. First, although he questions the Correspondence Postulate and wonders whether we could distin-guish causally relevant associations from associations that are reactions to the dream, he does not question the very heart of the postulate. That is, he does not ask how we know whether *any* of the associations to the dream are causally rele-vant. It would seem that he simply assumes this. But as we will later see, making this assumption is a very major and problematic step.

Second, even if we remain with Spence's more limited objection to the Correspondence Postulate, namely, that we do not know which of the associa-tions are relevant, we must ask once again why this objection should be limited to the dream. Do we not encounter the same difficulties with determining what is causally relevant when we come to the understanding of a fantasy we experi-enced a day ago? My critique here of Spence is not that he should have rejected the entire theory. My critique is, rather, that Spence is not making his point clear on why there is a problem that is specific to the dream (and not to other areas to which the psychoanalytic method is applied). His explicit intention is to do so and implicitly he distinguishes between the psychoanalytic method as applied to the dream and as it is applied to other areas. Only in relation to the dream does he require that there be clearly specified rules of transformation; only in relation to the dream is the limitation of the Correspondence Postulate disturbing to him. But Spence does not explain in what fundamental way the dream and other contexts are to be distinguished. He does not explain what warrants these special requirements specifically in relation to the dream. In the absence of such an explanation we are left with a general critique of psycho-analysis, rather than the specific critique that Spence is attempting to convey. Something is missing.

Grünbaum's Critique

Grünbaum's epistemological critique of Freud's dream theory directly refers to the dream as a unique context within psychoanalysis. His major statements regarding that theory appear in two chapters of his 1984 and 1993 books—"Repressed infantile wishes as instigators of all dreams: critical scrutiny of the compromise model of manifest dream content" (in 1984) and "Two new major difficulties for Freud's theory of dreams" (in 1993). In these chapters it is clear that he considers the dream to be distinguished by the very specific theory that Freud put forth regarding it. He suggests that Freudian dream theory is composed of two theses: (1) that the content of the dream is a fulfillment of a wish, and (2) that the dream's motive is an infantile repressed wish.

As in the case of Spence's critique, Grünbaum's both raises questions regarding the value of Freud's method of dream interpretation and also touches on issues related to what should be considered adequate criteria of justification, criteria that, according to Grünbaum, Freud fails to live up to. His major objections may be summarized as follows:

a. Freud's proof of his thesis that the motivational cause of the dream is a repressed wish rests on his method of free association, and was demonstrated primarily in his interpretation of the Irma dream. Grünbaum (1984) shows that the interpretation of that dream does not "authenticate free association as a trustworthy avenue for certifying that repressed infantile wishes are the formative causes of manifest dream content as claimed by Freud's theory" (p. 222). He does this by demonstrating that "the aggressive conscious wishes that Freud had on the day before his Irma dream were . . . patently fulfilled in [the dream's] . . . manifest content" (ibid.). Therefore, "free association played no excavating role in his recall of these wishes after the dream, for he had been avowedly conscious of them the evening before" (ibid.).

b. Freud maintains his wish-fulfillment theses only by way of ad hoc reasoning. Grünbaum illustrates how Freud would expand the interpretation until it would emerge as a wish-fulfillment. In one of the dreams (the dinner party dream—Freud, 1900, pp. 147–151) the dream appears to reflect the thwarting of the patient's wish. Freud then adds the auxiliary hypothesis that instead of being the patient herself, the person who figures in the dream is actually her rival. Freud brings further evidence to support this displacement, but Grünbaum considers this evidence faulty. This is intimately tied to his next criticism of Freud.

c. Grünbaum claims that Freud's evidence relies on the misguided assumption that associations to dream elements leading to a common thought (e.g., two associations implicating the dreamer's rival) warrant the conclusion that the common thought *caused* the dream elements. Citing Glymour's (1983) explication of this point, Grünbaum asserts that only the reverse can be affirmed—namely, that the dream elements caused the associations. This criticism parallels that of Spence.

d. The existence of counterwish dreams points to the falsity of Freud's theory, not only to its unfoundedness (as can be seen from the previous objections). Counterwish dreams are dreams that feature "the frustration of a wish or the occurrence of something clearly unwished-for" (Freud 1900, p. 157). In a nutshell, Grünbaum's argument is as follows: Freud brings an illustration of a dream in which the manifest content is clearly not a fulfillment of a wish, and in fact appears to be a direct contradiction of his theory. Freud concludes that the wish underlying the dream is the wish that he (Freud) be wrong. But, Grünbaum (1993) protests, if the manifest dream was indeed a contradiction of the dream theory, as Freud admits, then it "would be a bona fide—rather than only a prima facie or sham—refuting instance of the dream theory" (p. 364). In this case it is not only impossible to bring this dream as evidence of the wish-fulfilling nature of the dream—rather it contributes to the refutation of the theory that dreams are wish-fulfillments. Furthermore, Grünbaum (1993) adds, if the manifest content is to fulfill the wish that Freud be wrong, this could be done more directly: "For example, a public debate on the merits of Freud's own brand of psychoanalysis in which he is roundly defeated in arguments by some obscure Swiss scholar, who is a thin disguise for Carl Gustav Jung" (p. 366). Finally, he argues that for Freud to support his claim regarding the counterwish dream, he would have to show that indeed the two subclasses of people who should, in Grünbaum's view, dream such dreams—those who have a wish to prove Freud wrong and masochists—do indeed dream such dreams in a higher frequency than other dreamers. There is, Grünbaum claims, evidence to the contrary. For example, he himself had dreamt counterwish dreams prior to ever having read Freud. If Freud's claim regarding the meaning of the counterwish theory cannot be supported, if counterwish dreams do not result from the wishes that Freud postulates, is there then another kind of wish that is responsible for their appearance? If not, then one must ultimately simply conclude that there are dreams that run counter to Freud's theory.

     e. A necessary correlate of Freud's dream theory, were it true, would be the gradual decrease in quantity of dreams in individuals undergoing successful analyses. Given the parallel that Freud postulates between neurosis and dreaming, Freud's dream theory should predict a reduction in dream frequency among extensively psychoanalyzed patients. This is not the case and hence the theory is disproved.

     We may now turn to the examination of Grünbaum's critique. Any examination of Grünbaum's critique of Freud's dream theory must begin with his premise regarding what is "substantive" to that theory. As has been commonly recognized in relation to his portrayal of psychoanalysis in general, Grünbaum tends to confine very broad and mutually interwoven formulations to a single clearly defined "Master Proposition" that ultimately misses its mark (Wallerstein, 1986). Regarding the dream theory he argues that there are two main theses: the one referring to the wishful content and the other to the repressed infantile wish motive. As we will see later, these theses do not contradict what Freud professed, but are not so clearly formulated as Grünbaum presents them. It is not so clear that Freud was certain about the universality of the infantile origin of the dream (e.g., few of the dreams that Freud describes point to infantile origins, and Freud's remarks are at times tentative on this point), nor are these theses so strongly held by post-Freudians as Grünbaum claims (1984, p. 223).

More important, Grünbaum fails to see that one of Freud's most substantive and fundamental theses is the very fact of the dream being meaningful; the very fact that it is "a psychical structure which has a meaning and which can be inserted at an assignable point in the mental activities of waking life" (Freud, 1900, p. 1). For example, it is clear, that in the interpretation of the Irma dream it was not Freud's intent to prove a theory of repressed wish causation. It was his more immediate and direct intent to show that free association reveals that the dream has a meaning. By misportraying Freud's intention, Grünbaum leads up to the conclusion that free association failed at its task (point a), while in fact it failed only at the more specific task of revealing infantile wishes, but not at the task that more directly and explicitly interested Freud—discovering meaning.

Later Grünbaum (1984, p. 224) expressly recognizes this, but claims that Freud was actually employing here a complex strategy whereby he would authenticate (or, in the present terminology, justify) free association as a method that yields motives that engendered the dream, and then would "rest his substantive theory of dreams" (i.e., as universally wish-fulfilling, and as based on repressed infantile wishes) on the purportedly authenticated method. This hypothesis of Grünbaum's is in need of further substantiation. But in any case, it would seem that he considers it a trivial matter to justify the commonsense-psychology belief that the meaning of the dream can be understood in terms of the individual's motives that engendered them. In fact, however, as we will see later, the justification of this proposition, which lies at the heart of Freud's theory requires rather difficult maneuvers. For example, it is not at all obvious that a similarity between the motives that Freud experienced the night before the dream and the motives that are experienced within the dream warrants Grünbaum's conclusion that the one engendered the other. Grünbaum's trivialization of this point may be understood in terms of his singular focus on what he considers to be Freud's "substantive theory." This focus leads to the neglect both of Freud's concern with the very fact of the dream being a meaningful context influenced by the individual's motives and of the complex play with free association that is necessary in order to make the details of the dream meaningful. Ultimately, Grünbaum views the process of dream interpretation from a distance; he compares wishes and motives, but does not touch on the heart of the problem of the very meaningfulness of the dream, nor does he explore the intricacies that go into determining its meaning.

Grünbaum's second and third criticisms (points b and c) do indeed point to an important problem with Freud argumentation: the apparently ad hoc reasoning in Freud's interpretation of dreams. If, as Grünbaum believes, Freud is attempting to justify his theory of dreams by showing that it manages to make sense of some given dream, then his success is indeed questionable. With ad hoc reasoning, one may be able to retroactively explain dreams in virtually any way one wishes, thus failing to prove much. Admittedly, it often appears that this is the case; that Freud's proof of the validity of the dream theory rests on his repeated demonstration that dream interpretation reveals wishes. In these demonstrations Freud appears to be very atomistic in his method of justification: the meaning of each dream, and even of each feature in the dream, is supposedly shown to be validated on its own, independently of the rest of the psychoanalytic theory. It is therefore understandable that Grünbaum is led to assess Freud's theory in a similarly atomistic manner. Grünbaum singles out specific hypotheses (e.g., that the meaning of a specific dream is a wish) and applying an Atomistic Foundationalist model tests the justification of each such hypothesis in its own right. However there is room for alternative, non-atomistic forms of justification of the dream theory, some of which are to some degree implied in Freud's writings. Unfortunately, Grünbaum does not explore those alternatives. He does not go beyond the model of justification that Freud himself applied. He thus fails to see, as I willl ultimately show, that Freud's reasoning is not as ad hoc as it seems. If Freud's reasoning is seen as relying on the broader context of the psychoanalytic theory (contrary to Freud's own understanding of the basis of his reasoning), then it may be justified holistically; that is, the reasoning may be justified because it coheres with the larger theoretical context in which it is embedded.

Grünbaum's critique of Freud's assumption of the causal nature of associations (i.e., that the associations to the dream are what caused it) is equally damaging. I discussed this point earlier in the context of Spence's arguments. The difference here, however, is that in contrast to Spence, Grünbaum has no qualms about dispensing with the entire psychoanalytic theory. Grünbaum would not be disturbed in the least if the problems with associations to which he points turn out to be not special to the dream but rather to plague other aspects of Freud's theory as well. On the contrary, Grünbaum starts out from the premise that Freud's application of his method of associations to the discovery of meaning in the psychoanalytic context in general is without any foundation. When Grünbaum turns to the dream, his question is whether the method may be vindicated *at least* in this context. But it is important to recognize that it may be the case that once we start from the premise that the general psychoanalytic theory is flawed there remains no way to vindicate the dream theory. The dream theory may depend on the broader context of the general theory for its justification. This again touches on the possibility of justifying the dream theory atomistically, an issue that will come to the fore in the next chapter through a more comprehensive analysis of Freud's position.

The problematic effects of Grünbaum's general Atomistic approach is seen most clearly in his objection to Freud's hypothesis regarding the counterwish (point d). Grünbaum requires that Freud's hypothesis regarding the counterwish stand completely in its own right, independently of any other related theoretical conjecture (e.g., that the meaning of the dream is a wish). The question he poses is whether it can be shown, without reference to any other postulate, that when the content of a dream is the frustration of a wish, then it was caused by a wish of a specific kind. It may be seen here that Grünbaum's requirement is unduly strict and that his Atomistic form of justification is not the only legitimate form available. This requirement is equivalent to demanding of a geologist to explain any individual earthquake in its own terms, without using any general geological theory and independently of any knowledge gained elsewhere. As we have seen, there are Holistic forms of justification that would examine the counterwish hypothesis in the context of Freud's broader network of ideas on the dream and on psychoanalysis in general. It may turn out that given a broader theory of wish-fulfillment, Freud's seemingly ad hoc maneuvers in the context of his counterwish hypothesis—for example, the exceptions to the rule that he posits in order to avoid an apparent contradiction to his wish theory—are not ad hoc at all. It may be that as part of the broader context, they enhance the theory's coherence and help to better explain the data and in this sense to be justified, although in isolation they appear to lack support.

Another problem with Grünbaum's attack on Freud's counterwish proposition is that he seems to neglect the *details* of the broader wish-fulfillment theory. These must be taken into account in order to determine what could constitute a counterwish. Grünbaum (1993) seems to hold that, according to Freud, the thesis that the content of the dream is a wish means that "the manifest content must graphically display [a wish]—albeit in more or less disguised form" (p. 369). Therefore, when we come to test the counterwish hypothesis we should expect to see the counterwish most directly. Thus if there were a wish to refute Freud, it should have been directly expressed in a dream portraying him losing a debate with Jung. Furthermore, Grünbaum himself should be able to simply look at his dreams and note that they are of the counterwish variety. As we will see in the course of the close analysis of Freud, it is unclear how Grünbaum could have come to such a conclusion. Clearly Freud's theory does not imply that the wish should be there simply to be read off the dream. When Freud says that the content of a dream is a wish, he is referring to the fact that the latent thoughts that create the dream express a wish. These thoughts do not find direct expression in the dream; the dream is often absurd and the latent thoughts cannot be directly comprehended by the dreamer.

It would seem, furthermore, that it is Grünbaum's misguided view that wishfulness should be apparent in the manifest content (according to Freud) that leads him to reject the idea that in regard to the counterwish dreams Freud was speaking of "bona fide" contradiction, rather than only *apparent* contradiction. (One may add to this Grünbaum's tendency to read Freud in an overly literal way, neglecting the broader context of his remarks. If one takes Freud literally, he does in fact state that there seems to be a contradiction—albeit in the context of an obviously rhetorical question [Freud, 1900, p. 151].)

Similar neglect of the intricate nature of Freud's broader theory becomes apparent in the last of Grünbaum's arguments previously noted (point e)—namely, his argument that the necessary external support for the dream theory would be the reduction of frequency of dreaming among the well-analyzed. Here he is considering Freud's comments on the connection between dreams and neurosis in isolation from Freud's broader range of ideas on dreams. If the dream is like the neurosis, Grünbaum argues, then we should expect that the consequence of analysis will be the same in both cases. Both should result in the dissolution of the psychic structure. This conclusion is fallacious not only because despite the similarity there may be important differences, but also because Freud considered the dream in terms of relationships with a variety of phenomena, not only neurosis. For example, Freud said of the dream that it should be considered to be "a thought like any other." As such it would be rather strange to expect dissolution as the result of interpretation. Freud would not contend that the influence of latent contents would disappear as the result of analysis. We would not empty our unconscious as the result of our making our ideas conscious. This is basic to Freudian thought. Freud's ideas on the dream can be understood only within the broader network of ideas that he postulates. Grünbaum's attempts to single out certain ideas so that these could be empirically tested in isolation from the rest ultimately misrepresents what is essential to Freud's thinking.

It should be noted that Grünbaum does suggest that Freud in effect bases some of his theoretical ideas regarding the dream on other of his theoretical formulations. As just mentioned, he does point to the relationship that Freud posits between neurosis and dreaming. However, Grünbaum considers these to be extrapolations from one theory to the next, rather than considering them part of one overall theoretical network, and in this case he considers the extrapolation to be a mis-extrapolation. It is a mis-extrapolation both because the theory of neurosis is, according to Grünbaum, in itself a flawed theory, and because no attempt is made to seek external support for the dream theory, corresponding to the therapeutic improvement that was sought for the theory of neurosis.

Taken together, Grünbaum's critique correctly highlights certain limitations of Freud's justification of his dream theory. However, the numerous problems in his critique of Freud in this context reveal the great extent to which Grünbaum isolates specific propositions from that theory and then puts them to test independently of their theoretical context. This involves examining propositions regarding the dream not only in isolation from the broader psychoanalytic theory to which they belong, but also more immediately in isolation from the basic network of propositions of which Freud's dream theory is comprised. This not only limits the possibility of justification to a very Atomistic Foundationalist approach, but also distorts the essential nature of Freud's dream theory and the way he went about justifying it. Also, when Grünbaum does take note of the broader psychoanalytic frame in which the dream theory appears, his view that many of psychoanalysis' basic tenets are without any foundation limits the possibility of finding justification in a more Holistic form. For example, he does not allow for the possibility that the dream theory could find justification through its contribution to the broader theory, which in its turn may find its own support from the way its different subparts join together coherently and explain the data as a whole.

A Comparison of the Two Critiques

In Spence's critique the dream was considered a unique context—the general theory of psychoanalysis was in Spence's view immune to the criticisms he was raising in relation to the dream theory. It was unclear why. Grünbaum levels similar forms of criticism at the general theory and the dream theory alike. It is because he considers Freud's hypotheses regarding the dream to be different from those regarding his general theory that he sees a place to examine the justification of the dream theory independently. As we have seen, there were a variety of limitations to their expositions ranging from an overspecification of Freud's theses to a neglect of some of its most basic details. We also saw that neither Spence nor Grünbaum consider the justification of Freud's dream theory in the light of his broader theoretical propositions. Justification is considered very atomistically. Single propositions are studied in disregard to others, sometimes resulting in the distortion of their essential function and meaning. In Spence's case, extraordinarily rigorous criteria are set for the justification of these propositions.

These critiques highlight the necessity of an extensive study of Freud's arguments in favor of his dream theory. In order to examine the possibilities of justifying the dream theory we must have an in-depth understanding of its structure—both its internal structure and its place in relation to the broader theoretical network in which it is embedded. Before delimiting the nature of what is substantive to the theory and imposing on it a limited and rigorous set of criteria for its justification, we must see more precisely what exactly Freud claimed and how *he* went about justifying these claims. Through this we will come to a fuller understanding of the kinds of justification that are possible for the psychoanalytic theory of dreams.

CHAPTER TWO

Freud's Justification of His Dream Theory in The Interpretation of Dreams

No critic . . . can see more clearly than I the disparity arising from the problems and the answers to them; and it will be a fitting punishment for me that none of the unexplored regions of psychic life in which I have been the first mortal to set foot will ever bear my name or obey my laws.

—Freud to Fliess regarding *The Interpretation of Dreams,* in *The Complete Letters of Sigmund Freud to Wilhelm Fliess*

I can only express a hope that readers of this book will put themselves in my difficult situation and treat me with indulgence.

—Freud, *The Interpretation of Dreams*

The aim of this chapter is to explore the way in which Freud set forth his dream theory and attempted to justify it. A major question will be whether Freud has succeeded in adequately justifying the proposition that true meanings of the dream can be discovered through the application of the psychoanalytic method. As we will soon see, this proposition is, in fact, the heart of the psychoanalytic theory of dreams. Beyond the many facets of Freud's complex formulations regarding the dream, the processes involved in its formation, and the nature of the meanings that it contains, there is the very basic and essential claim that *the meaning of dreams can be actually discovered through an analytic process. It is the justification of this essential claim of the dream theory that I intend to examine.*

My examination will be a critical one in the sense that it will not rest on a priori assumptions regarding what Freud had said or how he justified it, but rather on a careful exposition of these. It will not take for granted—as often is the case in the psychoanalytic literature—that Freud's claim is true or justified. Rather the truth or justification of the claim is the subject matter of this study. I will follow Freud's argumentation, its structure, its correspondence to his intended structure of argumentation, its limitations, its relationship to empirical evidence, and the extent to which the evidence meets requirements acceptable to us today or to Freud then. My ultimate aim will be to evaluate whether Freud has succeeded in justifying his dream theory; whether Freud has indeed shown that the psychoanalytic method can lead to the discovery of the meaning of the dream. In striving toward this aim we may also come to understand the nature of the difficulties that are to be found in Freud's attempt at justification and the alternate routes that he could have taken to secure the foundation of his theory.

In this chapter my exploration of the way Freud justifies his dream theory will rely on Freud's presentation of his theory in *The Interpretation of Dreams*. This text is undoubtedly the most comprehensive and authoritative of Freud's statements regarding the dream. It is commonly agreed that in the breadth and depth of the exposition of the psychoanalytic understanding of the dream that it offers, the book has no rivals (e.g., Altman, 1969; Flanders, 1993; Rangell, 1987; etc.).[1] Freud himself maintained that beyond what was contained in that monumental book, little was ever added to the psychoanalytic theory of dreams (Freud, 1933a, p. 22). And it is well known that the major later innovations that were introduced were, for the most part, carefully inserted into it either as part of the text or as footnotes. However, the more significant consideration for me in choosing to focus specifically on this text is the fact that it contains the only comprehensive psychoanalytic attempt to justify the dream theory. Perhaps surprisingly, even today there are no other serious psychoanalytic attempts to justify this theory. Furthermore, the extensive illustrations and demonstrations of dream interpretations that Freud offers throughout the book make it particularly amenable to the uncovering of considerations that underlie the explicit statements regarding the way in which the theory was justified. In a few of his later writings Freud was to offer some additional partial arguments in favor of his theory. These additions will be discussed in chapter 4.

The Interpretation of Dreams comprises seven chapters of detailed formulations concerning the psychology of the dream. The first chapter is a review of the literature and the next six chapters address issues of method, wish-fulfillment, distortion, material and sources of the dream, dream work, and the psychology of the dream processes. It is possible to look at Freud's theory as a long series of independent statements: that dreams are motivated by wishes, that there is a latent dream thought, that the latent dream thought is distorted in several possible ways, that the distortion can be deciphered and the latent dream thought revealed by applying a certain technique, and so on. Indeed, gradually the psychoanalytic dream theory came to be commonly known in terms of such a list of propositions, with the primary one being that all dreams are wish-fulfillments. But in tracing the flow of Freud's thought as it unfolds in the course of the presentation of his ideas, it becomes apparent that such a schematization of Freud's ideas distorts and conceals essential aspects of his thinking. The nature of the relationship between Freud's ideas, and how they are intended to be supported and how they are actually supported, are integral to the understanding of his thinking. It is in the intricate tie between the flow of specific ideas and the Gestalt that they form that the essence of the Freudian dream theory, as well as its basis and justification, shine through. There is the danger that in breaking down the theory into independent statements, to the neglect of the careful analysis of their interrelationships, the essence of Freud's vision would be lost. A critical analysis of such statements would miss its mark and a more comprehensive understanding would be impossible. It is for this reason that in the present investigation I will focus on the inherent interrelationships of Freud's ideas. These emerge as one carefully traces the evolution of Freud's specific propositions. In the current study I will focus only on the first six chapters of *The Interpretation of Dreams*. These are the chapters that are most relevant to the issue of Freud's argument that the application of the psychoanalytic method can lead to the discovery of the meaning of the dream.

FREUD'S THREE PROPOSITIONS REGARDING THE MEANING OF DREAMS AND A PRELIMINARY ANALYSIS OF THE EPISTEMOLOGICAL PROJECT THAT HE FACES

The theory of dreams that Freud sets forth in *The Interpretation of Dreams* revolves around four basic propositions, three of which are directly relevant to the theory's essential core regarding the possibility of discovering meaning. In the following pages I will clarify the nature of these three propositions and discuss the kind of epistemological challenges that Freud will have to face when he comes to justify them. Later we will be able to see whether Freud does indeed meet these challenges.

The Propositions

Freud opens *The Interpretation of Dreams* with the following words:

> In the pages that follow I shall bring forward proof that there is a psychological technique which makes it possible to interpret dreams, and that, if that procedure is employed, every dream reveals itself as a psychical structure which has a meaning and which can be inserted at an assignable point

in the mental activities of waking life. I shall further endeavor to elucidate the processes to which the strangeness and obscurity of dreams are due and to deduce from those processes the nature of the psychical forces by whose concurrent or mutually opposing action dreams are generated. Having gone thus far, my description will break off, for it will have reached a point at which the problem of dreams merges into more comprehensive problems, the solution of which must be approached upon the basis of material of another kind. (Freud, 1900, p. 1)

In this opening paragraph we find a description of the essential propositions regarding dream theory that Freud intends to justify in the course of the book. It may be seen already at this very early point that Freud's basic initial thesis is not—as commonly believed—the simple assertion that dreams are wish-fulfillments. Rather what are at the center of his concern in relation to the dream are four basic propositions, three of which are stated explicitly. They are: (1) there is a technique that makes dream interpretation possible; (2) all dreams have meanings that in some specific way are related to the mental activity of wakeful life; (3) there are specific processes of obscuring the dream, the analysis of which reveals the psychic forces that generate the dream; and (4) (although not stated clearly here) there is a specific psychological model that underlies what is postulated in the previous statements. This latter proposition is discussed in chapter VII of Freud's book. It refers to the kind of psychological model that would have to be constructed in order to contain the findings that emerge regarding the discovery of the meaning of dreams. Since this proposition does not make a statement regarding the discovery of meaning but rather is *based* on findings regarding the discovery of meaning, it is not directly relevant to the purpose of the present study and will not be further discussed.

For the sake of clarity I will refer to the other three propositions as the "technique thesis," the "meaning thesis," and the "obscuration thesis." Together they encompass the basic theory that the dream contains meaning that may be discovered through the application of the psychoanalytic technique. It is important to recognize these theses because Freud's process of justification of the dream theory as a whole seems at times to take place through the justification of these separate theses.

The Epistemological Project

Careful study of the three relevant propositions points to the difficult challenges that will have to be met if Freud is to succeed in justifying his dream theory. In the course of their study the complex underlying interweaving nature of the propositions becomes apparent.

The "Technique Thesis" (There Is a Technique that Makes Dream Interpretation Possible):

The challenge. How can we find a criterion for the validity of the technique for the interpretation of dreams prior to knowing what the meaning of the dream is?

Obviously, it is possible to arbitrarily construct an indefinite number of techniques that will assign various meanings to any given dream. The question is how to determine whether any of these techniques yields the correct meaning of dreams. It should be recalled that we are here speaking of meaning in the actual causal sense of "meaning discovered." This is the sense in which Freud refers to meaning (see chapter 1). Thus the very fact that the technique yields interpretations would not be sufficient to support the claim that meanings have been arrived at. What would have to be shown is that the interpretations correspond to the actual meanings of the dream.

At first glance, Freud seems to be facing a problem of circularity. For it seems that in order to show that his technique produces correct interpretations of dreams, we need to know in advance what counts as "correct" interpretations; but in order to know the "correct" interpretations we need to use the technique.

To meet this challenge of circularity, Freud will have to either give us reasons for his technique that are independent of the interpretations that it produces; or, alternatively, show us how we can tell, before using the technique, which interpretations should count as the correct ones. The latter may be done either by supplying us with some general criterion for correctness, or alternatively through supplying us with dream interpretations that are not derived from the technique and that are known to be true. In other words, for Freud to respond to his challenge and prove the validity of his technique there are three possible routes. Route A: He must show that independently of the application of the technique, he knows the actual specific meaning of dreams, or at least of one dream. Although it is not at all clear how such independent knowledge of the meaning of dreams could possibly be available, if it were, the technique could then be justified through the examination of its capacity to arrive at this specific meaning (e.g., the specific wish). Route B: He must show that he knows of a formal characteristic that signifies that the correct meaning of the dream has been determined. The technique could then be justified through the examination of its capacity to elicit this characteristic (e.g., intelligibility, the demonstrated causal origin, some omen that indeed the dream was correctly interpreted, etc.). Route C: He must present strong arguments that the technique is correct independently of the results. According to this strategy there is no necessity in directly demonstrating that the technique elicits the true meaning.

The "Meaning Thesis" (All Dreams Have Meanings that in Some Specific Way are Related to the Mental Activity of Wakeful Life)

The challenge. How can the meaning thesis be justified prior to having proven the validity of the technique for discovering meaning?

Here we encounter the converse challenge to the previous one regarding the "technique thesis." While in that first thesis Freud had to justify the validity of his technique without relying in advance on the interpretations that it produces, here he has to say something about the interpretations without relying in advance on his technique. Specifically, in his present "meaning thesis" Freud states that meanings of dreams are of a certain kind—they are related to the psychic activity of wakeful life. Freud probably does not intend this thesis to be simply an assumption that is built in, and presupposed by his technique of interpretation. Rather, it seems that he intends it to be a separate thesis, over and above the "technique thesis." The problem is that in order to know that the "meaning thesis" is correct, (i.e., that meanings of dreams are indeed related to wakeful life), we need to determine meanings of dreams. But in order to determine meanings of dreams and see whether they are indeed related to wakeful life, it would seem that we need to have some technique for interpreting dreams. Thus it is unclear how the meaning thesis can be justified as a thesis that is separate from the technique thesis. Furthermore, if the meaning thesis rests on the technique, we need to know that the technique is valid; and the question is how to assess the validity of this technique without circularity, that is, without knowing in advance that the meanings that it produces are the correct ones.

What we are encountering here is the complex mutual intertwinement of Freud's propositions regarding technique and meaning. There seems to be some mutual dependence of the two that must be overcome for Freud to justify his theory without getting caught in circular reasoning. It is clear from the opening passage that Freud does not intend to be involved in such reasoning. On the contrary, from the way he posits these two theses his intentions seem to be to justify the technique independently of any knowledge regarding meaning and then to apply the technique to the discovery of the dream's meaning. He did not think that he would have to know or assume something regarding meaning in order to justify the technique, or to know or assume something regarding the technique in order to justify the claim that he is discovering meaning.

The "Obscuration Thesis" (There are Specific Processes of Obscuring the Dream, Their Analysis Reveals the Psychic Forces that Generate the Dream)

The challenge. Can the obscuring processes and the underlying generating forces be discoveries? Is this thesis not merely a reiteration of the "technique thesis" since technique and obscuration are inverted processes? Can psychic forces be discovered through the analysis of the obscuring processes that are not already known through the application of the technique?

It seems that in this thesis Freud intended two propositions: One, that the *processes* obscuring the dream are of a certain kind, and the other, that from an analysis of these processes the *psychic forces* generating the dream could be revealed. As Freud expands on the matter of dream processes it does appear that this is what he meant.

Regarding the obscuring processes, Freud is basically stating here that he has discovered the nature of the path that the dreamer's underlying meaning traverses in the course of its becoming the manifest dream. Clearly such a discovery would be very important to the justification of his claim that the meaning of the dream can be discovered. However, here too there may be seen to be a problematic interdependence between the "obscuration thesis" and the "technique thesis"—which in turn seems to depend on the "meaning thesis." It would seem that by determining the technique of interpreting dreams one is thereby determining the nature of the obscuring processes and vice versa; just as, to use a linguistic analogy, by determining the process of encoding a message one is thereby determining the method for decoding it and vice versa. A linguist can claim to have discovered the technique for decoding a military code into English, or alternatively to have discovered how to encode English messages into this military code, but he cannot reasonably claim to have discovered two separate things: *both* a technique for decoding *and* the process of encoding. The two are merely the same road traveled in opposite directions. Similarly, if one's technique is based on the postulation or discovery of certain relationships between what appears in the dream and its underlying meaning, then nothing really new could be introduced from then taking the underlying meaning that emerges from the application of that technique and comparing it with or relating it to what originally appears in the dream.

What is said here regarding the obscuring processes is also true regarding the possibility of discovering the psychic forces that generate the dream. The discovery of the psychic forces generating the dream is not independent of the application of the technique for finding the meaning of the dream, since for Freud to discover meaning *is* to uncover the underlying psychic processes. For example, to analyze the obscuring processes in a dream and find wish-fulfillment as the dream's underlying psychic force *is* to apply the technique for deciphering the meaning of the dream.

The conclusion is that the technique for finding the meaning the dream, the analysis of obscuring forces, and the discovery of the psychic forces generating the dream do not seem to be three different things but three ways of looking at the same idea. For the obscuration thesis to contain something additional to the technique and meaning theses, the process of analyzing obscuring processes or of discovering underlying psychic forces has to be shown to contain an independent element that is not already included in the application of the technique for finding the meaning of the dream. Without such independence Freud's "obscuration thesis" faces the danger of being only an *apparent* discovery, and as such of failing to serve as an additional contribution to the tenability of his claim regarding the discoverability of meaning in the dream.

Interim Conclusion Regarding Freud's Propositions

As we have seen, Freud's outline of his basic propositions was set forth as a series of independent propositions whose truth he was planning to demonstrate step-by-step. He claimed that he would show that he has a valid technique, the application of the valid technique will reveal true meaning, and the analysis of the true meaning will point to the obscuring processes as well as to the nature of the psychic force that generates the dream. But a preliminary analysis of the meaning of the propositions—independently of how Freud proceeds to examine and test them—points to an implicit network of interdependent ideas. Since the different propositions seem to complexly depend on each other, it would not be valid to use one of them to justify the tenability of the other. What would be needed is evidence that would point to the independence of his theses or provide some other solution to the problem of circularity. Whether Freud succeeds in meeting this epistemological challenge remains to be seen. An answer to this question emerges from the careful and detailed examination of Freud's justification of his propositions. I turn now to this examination.

FREUD'S JUSTIFICATION OF HIS PROPOSITIONS REGARDING THE
MEANING OF DREAMS

In a letter to Fliess Freud presents the basic structure of his intended argument in support of his propositions:

> The whole thing is planned on the model of an imaginary walk. At the beginning, the dark forest of authors (who do not see the trees), hopelessly lost on wrong tracks. Then a concealed pass through which I lead the reader—my specimen dream with its peculiarities, details, indiscretions, bad jokes—and then suddenly the high ground and the view and the question: which way do you wish to go now? (Freud, 1985, p. 365)

More specifically, Freud's plan emerges as follows:

a. To review the extant literature in order to show that the question of how to interpret the dream is not resolved, that the scientific focus is on its being a somatic event and hence meaningless, and that such explanations do not explain the phenomenon of the dream, especially not the specific form the dream takes. That is, the existent explanations underdetermine the dream.

b. To apply his technique of analysis developed through his work with neuroses to the analysis of one of his dreams ("the specimen dream") and to show that through the application of this technique the underlying meaning of the dream emerges (the "technique thesis").

c. Once the nature of the meaning of Freud's one dream is revealed to be of a specific kind—a wish-fulfillment—Freud wants to show that indeed this finding is generalizable to all dreams (the "meaning thesis"). Here his argument rests on the evidence of (1) dreams that are obviously wish-fulfillments and (2) dreams that appear not to be wish-fulfillments but ultimately can be demonstrated through their analysis to be wish-fulfillments.

d. Through the comparison of the dream in its manifest form with the wishful dream thought that emerges through the correct interpretation, Freud deduces the processes that underlie the distortion of the dream as well as the motives for this distortion. Here Freud puts forth his ideas on the nature of the dream work, as well as his ideas on dream censorship defending against unconscious thoughts (the "obscuration thesis").

As we noted regarding Freud's presentation of his three propositions, here too, as he presents his basic line of intended argumentation, he does not seem to be aware of or deal with the basic problem of the interdependence of his three propositions regarding the meaning of the dream. He presents his "imaginary walk" as one that is intended to simply proceed linearly. There is no mention of the potential circular reasoning. We will now see whether this linear process of justification that Freud outlines here can actually be carried out to a successful conclusion.

As we turn from Freud's intentions to the nature of the arguments that he *in effect* puts forth in the course of his book, it is important to note that they are not always immediately apparent. While Freud tries to follow his intended line of argumentation, the arguments themselves can often be discerned only through a difficult process of teasing them out. This involves sifting through Freud's long and detailed illustrations to extract the underlying theoretical foundations, and being attuned to the logic of his statements without being distracted by the lure of Freud's friendly and charming prose. What emerges from this effort is a complex picture. At times it is even difficult to distinguish between the propositions, arguments, hypotheses, and assumptions, and between what was proven and what remains to be proven.

A blatant example of this complexity may be seen already at the beginning of Freud's second chapter. There he states: "Interpreting a dream implies assigning a 'meaning' to it—that is, replacing it by something which fits into the chain of our mental acts as a link having a validity and importance equal to the rest" (Freud, 1900, p. 92). Freud is here referring not to the act of interpreting but to the state of having arrived at a true interpretation. In our analysis of the propositions Freud put forth at the opening of his book we saw that his second proposition, his "meaning thesis," considered such a "fitting into the chain of mental events" to be a *discovery* regarding the nature of the meanings that the dream could contain. Here it is presented as part of an a priori *definition* of meaning in the context of the dream. Freud here informs the reader that, in his view, the act of interpreting will be completed when the dream is found to have a meaning of this specific kind—one that fits in with our mental acts of wakefulness—and that to find that dreams have meaning is to find that dreams have meaning of this specific kind. This is a very significant shift. Freud here places constraints on the specific nature of the dream's meaning. In so doing he begs the question he wished to answer regarding the specific nature of the dream's meaning. He seems to be saying that only when the interpretation process yields meaning of the specific kind can this process be considered to have revealed the dream's meaning. But why should this be the case? Freud offers no explanation of this seemingly arbitrary maneuver, nor does he even seem to recognize that a significant maneuver is here being made, for he makes no special note of it.

Moreover, in these definitions of "interpretation" and "meaning" Freud introduces a great deal of unclarity into the structure of his argument. For example, he does not specify whether in these definitions he is referring to sufficient or necessary conditions for meaning. Is he suggesting that the sufficient criteria for having interpreted the dream correctly is the very fact that it is "replac[ed] . . . by something which fits into the chain of our mental acts as a link having a validity and importance equal to the rest" (ibid.) or is he only suggesting that such "fitting in" is a minimal necessary condition for there to be meaning? Can we indeed conclude that any content that fits into the chain of our mental acts may be considered to be a meaning of the dream? If this is Freud's intention, then this is a very crucial point. It directly pertains to the issue of Freud's strategy of justification, for it suggests that Freud heavily relied on a specific kind of coherence in this context: When what underlies the dream fits in well with the thoughts of wakeful life, then we are justified in assuming that we have arrived at the meaning of the dream.

In the course of Freud's presentation of his argument in favor of his dream theory, such indirect and confusing statements and maneuvers often infiltrate his line of thinking. My following systematic presentation of Freud's arguments is the result of an ardent endeavor to bring to light both Freud's manifest argument and his implicit ideas that clearly play a role in his attempt to justify his dream theory.

The Literature Review

Freud read and wrote about the available literature on dreams (with considerable reluctance and unpleasure) because he believed that such a review would be important to the acceptance of his book in scientific circles (Freud, 1985, p. 365). The primary explicit use of the literature review in the course of his argument in favor of his dream theory is to show that available approaches to the dream do not adequately explain the phenomenon of the dream. That is, that the various theories, such as those that view the dream as a transformation of certain somatic phenomena, fail to explain the specific forms that the dream takes; they fail to explain, for example, the specific memories that are invoked in the course of the transformation. Freud seems to suggest that the theories not only underdetermine the dream but they also leave unexplained the contradictory findings of the different writers. For example, how is it that the images in the dream are all traceable to the past (according to one writer) and yet related to present-day events (according to another)? The conclusion that Freud leads us to here is that there is room and necessity for a new dream theory that will explain the phenomena and the contradictions that have been left unresolved.

The literature review may, however, be seen to play a more direct and important part in Freud's epistemological project. Through his extensive review (he devotes approximately one hundred pages of his six-hundred-page book to it), Freud shapes the nature of the explanandum in a way that prepares the ground for his new propositions and implicitly provides them with support. His presentation of the theories and the data that they have come to explain is such that one not only feels the absence of a theory that would explain more, but also the absence of a theory of a very specific kind. The presentation of the literature forebodes his later formulations. Moreover, it lends legitimacy to certain assumptions that underlie his formulations but that go unnoted and unsupported in his presentation of the formulations themselves.

I will explain this through an illustration: In his review, and based on the available literature, Freud accepts as a fact the idea that "All the material making up the content of a dream is in some way derived from experience, that is to say, has been reproduced or remembered in the dream" (Freud, 1900, p. 11). To use Freud's own words: "We may regard this as *undisputed* fact" (ibid., italics my own). But this fact is clearly in dispute. Freud himself notes this but a few pages earlier. He quotes Burdach (1838), Fichte (1864), and Strumpell (1877) as writers who maintain views that contradict the previous one. They hold that "In dreams, daily life with its labours and pleasures, its joys and pains, is never repeated" (Burdach, 1838, p. 499, cited in Freud, 1900, p. 7). Or even more explicitly Freud states: "The contradiction between these two views upon the relation between dream-life and waking life seems in fact insoluble" (Freud, 1900, p. 9). In this discrepancy in Freud's reporting we find him latently securing a foundation for his propositions regarding the dream. The "undisputed fact" that the dream material is part of daily experience provides a basis for the later claim that all dreams have meanings that in some specific way are related to the mental activity of wakeful life (the "meaning thesis"). And yet the simultaneous reference to the contradiction between dream life and waking life points to the fact that these daily experiences must have undergone some form of transformation (the "obscuration thesis"). In subsequent chapters, when Freud begins to more directly justify his theoretical formulations, he indeed takes as a given the personal experiential source of the dream, and at the same time points to the value of the theory, in that it can explain what he believes to be an apparent contradiction between this given fact and the fact that the dream describes events quite foreign to daily experience. Thus in shaping the data in the way that he does, Freud eases the path to the justification of his propositions. The problem is, however, that it is not at all clear that in this shaping the phenomenon of the dream is being fairly represented. Freud's own literature review suggests that it is not.

Freud's review of the literature contains many additional instances of such problematic presentation of the data and theories, with the implicit aim of securing the ground for his own theoretical propositions. Some outstanding instances can be found in Freud's remarks on (1) the dream as comprised of fragments ("Dreams yield no more than *fragments* of reproductions: and this is so general a rule that theoretical conclusions may be based on it" [Freud, 1900, p. 21]); (2) the dream as images ("what are truly characteristic of dreams are only those elements of their content which behave like images" [p. 50]); (3) the dream as transformations of ideas (Freud here makes an unnoted shift from the view that in the dream a hallucination *replaces* ideas, to the view that in the dream a hallucination *transforms* them, ibid.); (4) there being only two alternatives emerging from the literature: either to deny the possibility of further and more specifically tracing the causes of the dream, or to assume that there are additional causes to be elucidated. (This puts aside the possible position that there may be additional causes to elucidate but that they are beyond our capacity to trace [p. 29]); and (5) how all apparently different kinds of dreams are essentially similar in regard to the basic question of their having meaning (as evidenced by the fact that all the different researchers seem to hold the "conviction that some distinguishing feature *does* exist, which is universally valid in its essential outline" [ibid.]).

These smuggled suppositions obviously do not prove the truth of Freud's propositions regarding the dream, but it may be seen that they do make the propositions more reasonable. The first two instances indirectly provide support for the "technique thesis," the third instance for the "obscuration thesis," and the last two for the "meaning thesis." Once again the problem is that it is not at all clear how Freud can justify his portrayal of the literature and its implications.

Many of the points that Freud refers to are in dispute and it is not even always clear how one would go about resolving the dispute conclusively (e.g., regarding what is the *most* essential characteristic of the dream). And yet some of the disputes seem to simply disappear within Freud's unusual integrations or reformulations.

Ultimately one must put in question the value of Freud's literature review to the justification of his dream theory. The support for his propositions that the review indirectly provides is based on what clearly appears to be illegitimate reorganization of the data and questionable inferences drawn therefrom.

The Technique

Following the first step in Freud's plan, namely the literature review, Freud now intends to move on to the second step of applying his technique of analysis to dreams. Although the journey through the "dark forest of authors (who do not see the trees)"—as Freud refers to the reader's encounter with the literature review (Freud, 1985, p. 365)—may not be *essential* to Freud's argument in favor of his dream theory, the journey through "the concealed pass" (ibid.) is. That is, while the review of the literature is aimed at making the reader favorably inclined toward the ideas that Freud is to put forth, at easing the presentation of these ideas, and providing indirect support for them, it is not directly essential or necessary for his line of argument. In contrast, what is essential to Freud's argument is what underlies and emerges from his application of his technique of analysis to one of his dreams. Here Freud conducts what he refers to as an "experiment" (Freud, 1900. p. 105). He applies the technique of analysis that he developed through his work with neuroses, to one of his dreams, his "specimen dream." According to Freud's strategy of justification, in order for him to justify his "technique thesis," he must demonstrate here that the application of this technique to the dream results in the discovery of the dream's meaning. Here lies "the concealed pass." Freud's experiment is a crucial step in his attempt to justify his dream theory. In order to understand and evaluate Freud's justification it is important to understand the design of this experiment and see whether it indeed succeeds or fails to show that the underlying meaning of the dream emerges.

Freud develops his ideas in this context in the following way.

a. He states that a technique of interpretation exists that has not yet been generally applied to the interpretation of the dream. This is a factual statement. Freud points to the two popular techniques of interpreting dreams—symbolic interpretation and decoding—and reveals their limitations. He then turns to an alternative technique. This is the technique of free association that he applied to the understanding of the neurotic symptoms or psychopathological structures of his patients. In his brief description of the technique Freud's emphasis is on the suppression of the critical faculty that must be brought about so that additional material may come into consciousness. He mentions that this material is then to be interpreted, but he does not specify the details of the process (Freud, 1900, p. 100).

b. He states that he has applied this technique of interpretation to the dream: In listening to the associations of the neurotic patient to his symptoms or pathological ideas, Freud noted that reports of dreams were inserted into the psychic chain. "It was then only a short step to treating the dream itself as a symptom and to applying to dreams the technique of interpretation that had been worked out for symptoms" (Freud, 1900, p. 101). As a description of what he and his patients did, this too is a statement of fact.

However, it remains somewhat unclear whether in speaking of it being "only a short step to treating the dream . . . as a symptom" Freud is referring only to a descriptive level, whether he is simply describing the way in which he came across his technique. A more likely possibility is that he is here speaking of an inferential step in the context of justification. That is, the "short step" refers to Freud's position that the dream is a psychic product that is not very far off from the symptom in terms of some essential characteristics and therefore it is legitimate to treat the dream as though it were a symptom. If this is what Freud means, then his statement is problematic. In this latter inferential sense, it is a statement regarding the justification of the technique as a method for the discovery of meaning in the dream. Freud, however, does not provide any adequate evidence in support of this inference. Clearly, the very fact that dreams were inserted into the neurotic's chain of associations is not sufficient in this regard. Were a patient to introduce into the chain of associations mathematical equations, a piece of poetry, or a recollection of some event that occurred in the course of the day, we may assume that Freud would not have treated these as symptoms.

In the absence of some additional support of what appears to be Freud's inferential step we cannot legitimately consider Freud's statement regarding the application of his technique to the dream to be anything more than an anecdotal description of how he had chosen the technique that he applied to the dream. We cannot regard the statement as a contribution to the justification of the technique, even though it may misleadingly appear to be such a contribution.

c. He states that in applying the technique to the dream, the dream must not be related to as "a whole," but rather must be considered in terms of fragments into which it can be broken down. The "must" here seems at first to be of a pragmatic nature. Freud explains that the dream must be cut into fragments ("I put the dream before him cut up into pieces") in order to elicit associations to it; when requested to associate to the dream as a whole the dreamer comes up with a blank (Freud, 1900, p. 103). But Freud's position seems to be based on theoretical considerations as well. He implies, for example, that he "regards dreams from the very first as being of a composite character, as being conglomerates of psychical formations" (p. 104). Although this remark may be only a *description* of one consequence of his pragmatically derived maneuver of fragmenting the dream, it seems more like a *theoretical* explanation, a rationale for the maneuver. It explains why cutting up the dream into pieces is justified, why patients tend to have associations to the dream only when it is cut up in this way.

It may be seen that neither the pragmatic explanation nor the theoretical one can be considered to be good explanations of this statement regarding the necessity of fragmenting the dream. The fact that fragmenting the dream is useful for eliciting associations does not necessarily make it a good step for discovering the meaning of the dream. The theoretical explanation, on the other hand, is presented axiomatically. It defines the nature of the dream ("as being conglomerates of psychical formations") without reason or evidence. (Here we may see an example of how Freud's literature review—from which Freud sums up that "Dreams yield no more than *fragments* of reproductions" [Freud, 1900, p. 21]—provides an illusion of support. It attenuates the reader's possible discomfort at this unsubstantiated theoretical statement.)

Thus, as in the case of Freud's previous statement, we cannot consider the present statement to be one that contributes to the justification of the application of his technique to the dream. It merely describes what Freud did. He considered the dream in terms of fragments rather than relating to it as a whole. While Freud seems to imply that there was good reason for this maneuver, ultimately the reasons he presents are far from sufficient.

d. He proposes putting his technique to the test by seeing whether it allows for the interpretation of one of his own dreams. Freud here presents in detail the analysis of his "Irma dream," the dream that he refers to as his "specimen dream." His analysis leads him to the conclusion that through this technique he indeed arrived at its interpretation, at its hidden meaning. According to Freud, this has implications both for the technique and the meaning of dreams. Not only is the technique that was previously reserved for the study and treatment of pathology now to be considered an appropriate one for dream analysis, but also now that such a technique is found, information is made available concerning the kinds of meanings that may be hidden within the dream.

An Important Note on Freud's Independent Criteria for Demonstrating the Validity of His Technique

It is very important to note at this point that in putting his technique to test in the interpretation of his particular dream, *Freud does not explicitly put forth what he considers to be the criteria that would indicate its validity, but that two implicit criteria emerge in the course of the analysis—the intelligibility or coherence of the overall meaning, and the reasonableness of the interpretative steps.* It may be seen that up to the interpretation of the "specimen dream," Freud's statements have not provided any real support for the *general* validity of the technique as a method that would lead to the discovery of meaning in the dream. His statements (a, b, c) regarding the existence of the technique, that it may be applied to the dream, and the fact that it has been applied to the dream, were revealed to be insignificant in terms of justifying his contention that it is indeed appropriate to apply this technique to the dream; that it can lead to true meanings of the dream. Hence the demonstration of the validity of the technique now depends on the outcome of his application of it to a *particular* dream, his "specimen dream." But how does Freud plan to go about demonstrating this?

To recall, there were three possible routes to showing that the technique indeed leads to the discovery of the meaning of the dream: Freud must either know the meaning of the dream in advance and show that the technique reveals this meaning, or he must know of some formal characteristic that indicates that the meaning of the dream has been discovered and show that his interpretation process elicits this characteristic, or finally he must present arguments showing that in applying his technique he is interpreting the dream correctly, independently of the results. In the course of his interpretation of the "specimen dream," Freud does not specify the routes that he chooses, but he seems to be relying on the latter two. When he comes to a comprehensive understanding of all the aspects of the dream, when they all fit together, only then does he consider the dream analysis successful. It is here that we see a latent expression of reliance on the second route. That is, if the technique yields a coherent and intelligible picture, then we may know that the meaning has been attained. This reliance on coherence and intelligibility as the formal characteristic indicative of the discovery of the dream's meaning is in line with Freud's remark, cited earlier, that "[i]nterpreting a dream implies assigning a 'meaning' to it—that is, replacing it by something which fits into the chain of our mental acts as a link having a validity and importance equal to the rest" (Freud, 1900, p. 92). Freud seeks comprehensive coherence as a sign of having discovered the dream's meaning.

Freud's choice of the third route is also expressed in a latent form. It may be seen through his pervasive attempts to argue that his numerous interpretive steps leading up to the discovery of the dream's meaning are reasonable, or even inevitable. He is not concerned here with demonstrating the value of the end-product of the interpretive process, but rather with convincing the reader that each step of his interpretive process was legitimately taken. He aims to show that each move is correct regardless of the results of the process.[2]

In choosing these routes Freud avoids the potential danger of circularity, which emerged in the earlier discussion of Freud's theses. He does not rely on knowing the meaning of the dream in advance, which would most likely entail having had some earlier valid technique for knowing this meaning, and thus would involve him in circular reasoning. Rather, Freud seeks some independent criteria for the technique. As we will later see, the choice of these independent criteria for the justification of his "technique thesis" renders Freud's other two theses (the "meaning" and the "obscuration" theses) superfluous. Considering them as independent theses indeed results in circular reasoning. They are, in fact, mere *derivatives* of the "technique thesis." Freud's essential dream theory collapses into one thesis regarding the possibility of discovering meaning through the application of his technique.

The crucial question that we now must address is whether Freud indeed succeeds in justifying this thesis along either of the two routes that he has chosen. After examining this question in the following pages, we will be able to return to the rest of Freud's arguments in favor of his dream theory.

Freud's Analysis of His "Specimen Dream"

The Text of the Dream. This is how Freud describes the dream:

Dream of July 23rd-24th, 1895

A large hall—numerous guests, whom we were receiving.—Among them was Irma. I at once took her on one side, as though to answer her letter and to reproach her for not having accepted my 'solution' yet. I said to her: 'If you still get pains, it's really only your fault.' She replied: 'If you only knew what pains I've got now in my throat and stomach and abdomen—it's choking me'—I was alarmed and looked at her. She looked pale and puffy. I thought to myself that after all I must be missing some organic trouble. I took her to the window and looked down her throat, and she showed signs of recalcitrance, like women with artificial dentures. I thought to myself that there was really no need for her to do that.—She then opened her mouth properly and on the right I found a big white patch; at another place I saw extensive whitish grey scabs upon some remarkable curly structures which were evidently modelled on the turbinal bones of the nose.—I at once called Dr. M., and he repeated the examination and confirmed it . . . Dr. M. looked quite different from usual; he was very pale, he walked with a limp and his chin was clean-shaven. . . . My friend Otto was now standing beside her as well, and my friend Leopold was percussing her through her bodice and saying: 'She has a dull area low down on the left.' He also indicated that a portion of the skin on the left shoulder was infiltrated. (I noticed this, just as he did, in spite of her dress.) . . . M. said: 'There's no doubt it's an infection, but no matter; dysentery will supervene and the toxin will be eliminated.' . . . We were directly aware, too, of the origin of the infection. Not long before, when she was feeling unwell, my friend Otto had given her an injection of a preparation of propyl, propyls . . . propionic acid . . . trimethylamin (and I saw before me the formula for this printed in heavy type) . . . Injections of that sort ought not be made so thoughtlessly. . . . And probably the syringe had not been clean. (Freud, 1900, p. 107)

Freud's analysis of the dream continues on pages 107–121. Since the details of the analysis cannot be summarized, I refer the reader to those pages. What follows here is a critique of some of the major steps Freud took in the course of the analysis.

A Critical Examination of Freud's Analysis in the Light of the Criteria of Each of the Two Routes. It is necessary to examine Freud's analysis of the "specimen dream" in the light of the two criteria that he implicitly relies on for the justification of his technique as a valid method for the discovery of the meaning of the dream: First, the formal characteristic of intelligibility or coherence that indicates that a correct meaning has been reached (Route B). Second, step-by-step arguments showing the correctness of the procedure of the dream-analysis (Route C). I will begin with the examination of the latter, since it appears chronologically first in Freud's presentation.

The question here is whether Freud's detailed process of analysis and the arguments that he brings forth for the various kinds of interpretative steps that he takes in its course reveal that indeed the technique that is being applied is appropriate. That is, independently of the ultimate result of the analytic process, whether Freud convincingly shows that he is taking the right path in carrying out the analysis in the way that he does. After presenting the problems with the way Freud carries out the analysis I will argue that he does not. I will then turn to the second route and to the criteria of intelligibility or coherence of the comprehensive meaning. Here we will take the process of dream interpretation as epistemologically arbitrary and inquire whether the end-product that it yields justifies it. The question will be whether in the case of dream interpretation of the kind Freud offers us, intelligibility can serve as a valid criterion of having discovered a true meaning of the dream. Here too my answer will be in the negative. Freud fails to justify his technique.

We may now turn to the details of the examination.

Problems with Freud's Process of Analysis (The Criterion Used for Route C). In the following pages I present some representative and illustrative examples of the basic kinds of problems that arise in the course of Freud's analysis of his "specimen dream." These raise questions as to whether Freud's interpretative steps are necessary, warranted, or even reasonable. It should be noted that the present list does not fully exhaust the numerous kinds of difficulties that emerge, and that there is at times overlap between the different categories of problems.

First there are problems with the determination of the context of meaning. Freud begins the process of applying his technique to the dream by delimiting a specific context in which the dream is to be viewed. This context implicitly allows for certain kinds of meanings to be assigned to the dream. No rationale for this highly consequential maneuver is offered. The maneuver involves two basic steps or kinds of problems.

Problem 1: The insertion of the dream into the ongoing meaningful events of life. This first step takes place in two stages. First Freud points to the existence of a causal connection between the dream and the events of the day preceding it, and then he posits that the connection is between the dream and the *meanings* of the events, not merely, the events themselves. Let us examine this step in greater detail.

Freud puts forth a preamble to the dream, which describes certain aspects of his interactions in reality with major characters of his dream: his patient Irma and his two friends and colleagues, Otto and Dr. M. The focus is on the events of the day prior to the dream, where Freud felt reproved by Otto for his treatment of Irma and consequently wrote up the case, intending to present it to Dr. M. in order to justify himself. Freud then describes the dream. Following this description and without any further argumentation Freud concludes:

> This dream has one advantage over many others. It was immediately clear what events of the previous day provided its starting point. My preamble makes that plain. The news which Otto had given me of Irma's condition and the case history which I had been engaged in writing till far into the night continued to occupy my mental activity even after I was asleep. (Freud, 1900, pp. 107–108)

The causal connection between the dream and the events of the previous day does *seem* to be immediately obvious. That is, it does seem likely that the events of the previous day caused the dream. However, if we are to treat this dream analysis as an "experiment," further evidence is required. While a positive tie is found between the figures preoccupying Freud's mind during the day prior to the dream and those preoccupying his mind during the dream itself, this is insufficient information to conclude that the one *caused* the other. For example, clearly data regarding the frequency of finding such positive ties would be essential. (In fact, Freud seems to imply in the above quotation, that at least on the manifest level such ties are infrequently found. If indeed that is the case, an instance of a positive tie would not be evidence of a causal relationship, even if it is a particularly impressive instance.)

Matters become more problematic as Freud moves on to suggest that the dream is caused not only by the manifest image of the events of the previous day, but specifically by their underlying meanings. He moves on to this suggestion after he presents the text of the dream. In his comments following its presentation Freud states that what caused the dream were not only his preoccupations with the characters in question during the day prior to the dream, but rather among its causes were also the *specific events within the interaction with these characters*—"the news which Otto had given me of Irma's condition and the case history which [I] had been engaged in writing." The text of the dream itself does not refer directly either to the news or the case history.

What Freud is saying here is that what caused the dream and what is reflected through it are not only the images of people or of the events with whom or with which he was preoccupied the previous day, but rather what these *images* represented, the place they held for him or what they "*meant*" to him, specifically in the interaction he had with these images the previous day. This basically involves two propositions. Firstly, that the dream is affected by the meanings contained, or represented, by the assumed causal object. That is, the image of Otto in the dream contains or represents elements of who Otto is for Freud when awake, or that the meaning of the event with Otto is preserved in the dream. It is not simply that the image of Otto or of the event causes the image of these in the dream. The second proposition entailed here is that some of the most effective or influential meanings tied to the assumed causal object (Otto) are those that were prominent at the time of the last appearance of the causal object. That is, the dream is affected not only by who Otto is for Freud when awake, but also—at least in part—by who Otto was at the moment at which the causal process began. In sum, Freud suggests that Otto's image the previous day *caused* the appearance of Otto's image at night, and that that image represented or *meant* who Otto was in general for Freud, but *most* specifically that image represented or meant who Otto was for him on the previous day, (i.e., the bearer of the news regarding Irma's condition).

Even were we to grant Freud the causal connection between a preoccupation with Otto during the day and during the dream, we would still have difficulty with these meaning connections. Clearly, Freud does not contend (as is immediately apparent from his subsequent remarks) that *all* objects in dreams are connected to objects in wakeful life by reflecting the same underlying meaning on both occasions. Were Freud never to have seen Otto before in his life, then it would not be the meaning of Otto for Freud that was being represented in the dream, for there would not exist any such direct meaning. And if it is *possible* for an object to exist in a dream in such a way that it is unrelated to its immediate meaning in reality, it is then equally possible that even when the object in the dream does correspond to an object that exists in reality, it may not represent the meanings that the individual ascribes to that object in actuality. It would be necessary for Freud to show that the appearance of the object in the dream is not only causally determined by the object of wakeful life, but indeed is accompanied at times by some of the meanings actually ascribed to it in wakeful life. Furthermore, he would have to show that the meanings that appear in the dream are those that are relevant to the event that caused the dream. It is possible, for example, that the image of Otto during the day set off an image of Otto during the dream, and that in the dream the image contained meanings of who Otto was for Freud (e.g., a friend, a colleague, a doctor, etc.), but that it did not contain anything of the meanings of Otto specifically from the encounter that Freud claims had caused the appearance of Otto's image in the dream. That is, the appearance of Otto's image in the dream may have had nothing to do with the reality of Otto as bearer of the news regarding Irma's condition.

Freud brings no evidence or arguments to support these initial general contentions that he puts forth regarding the existence of such causal and meaningful connections between wakeful life and the dream.[3] He asserts that recognizing these connections does not yet allow one to understand the dream. ("Nevertheless, no one who had only read the preamble and the content of the dream itself could have the slightest notion of the what the dream meant, I myself had no notion" [p. 108].) But in pointing to the connections between the preamble and the dream Freud is, in a very significant way, determining and delimiting the dream's context of meaning. He is inserting the dream into the ongoing meaningful events of life. It is within this context that he carries out his further analysis of the dream in an attempt to discover its specific meaning.

Problem 2: The fragmentation of the dream into sections that arouse associations in the dreamer. Earlier we noted that Freud referred to a combination of pragmatic and theoretical reasons why the dream should be fragmented before analysis rather than examined as a whole. We had found the reasons unconvincing. As Freud turns to the actual analysis of his "specimen dream," it seems that he supports this idea of fragmenting by a further and more specific theoretical assumption concerning the fragments of the "psychical formations" that come together to form the dream. The assumption is that these pieces of "psychical formations" find expression in the dream such that they correspond to a fragment of the manifest dream, and that this fragment is defined by the fact that it arouses associations in the dreamer when the dreamer in wakefulness reexamines the dream. For example, the word "dysentery" (which appears in Freud's dream) is a source of associations, while the word "injection" (also in the dream) is not. Freud assumes, therefore, that the fragment "dysentery" conceals a "psychical formation," a meaningful thought, which may be accessed through the associations it evoked. That is, Freud believes that an underlying thought finds expression in this fragment because it aroused associations. Clearly, were Freud to demand from himself associations to the word "injection" he may have some. But Freud would not consider such "forced" associations to be relevant. In order to arrive at the underlying thoughts of which the dream is composed it is necessary, according to Freud, to cut the dream according to the pieces of the dream that naturally arouse associations.

Freud does not make explicit the fact that, in effect, he is fragmenting the dream according to a certain method. He does not specify his implicit criteria according to which this fragmentation is done. In line with this, no rationale for this kind of fragmentation is offered. Implicit is the theoretical notion that there are underlying thoughts that correspond to association-arousing pieces of the dream. But what is the basis for this notion? Indeed, why should it be that this technique of fragmentation is the one that cuts the dream at its joints, so to speak? The answers to these questions are not at all self-evident. There is no apparent reason to believe that specifically this technique—convenient as it may be in terms of eliciting associations—is the one that leads to whatever meanings went into the making of the dream, rather than an alternative technique, such as one that cuts the dream at every sentence, for example, or at every word. Thus, while in fragmenting the dream in this way the dream's basic context of potential meaning is further qualified, and while an additional constraint on the nature of the dream's meaning is introduced, the justification for this move remains unclear.[4]

We come now to a second cluster of problems in Freud's attempt to justify the analysis of his dream. Here I refer to *problems in the determination of specific meanings.* Having to some extent determined the basic meaningful context in which the dream is to be viewed, Freud now turns to determine the dream's specific meanings. Here we encounter the heart of the difficulties with Freud's application of his technique. These can be divided into three broad categories: Freud's reliance on assumptions that he set out to prove, his neglect of important qualitative differences between different kinds of associations, and his introduction of arbitrary maneuvers.

Problem 3: Freud's reliance on assumptions which he originally set out to prove. Two primary assumptions are involved. The first assumption is that *statements contained within fragments are sensible and realistic.* Freud does not directly state that he is making this assumption. The fact that he is indeed making it, however, becomes apparent from the study of what it is within each fragment that he finds necessary to explain. For example: In his associations to Irma's pains Freud says that "pains in the stomach were among my patient's symptoms but were not very prominent . . . I wondered why I decided upon this choice of symptoms in the dream?" (Freud, 1900, p. 109). Or, in his associations to her pale and puffy look, he writes: "My patient always had a rosy complexion. I began to suspect that someone else was being substituted for her" (ibid.). This kind of inquiry continues throughout. Explanation is required when there is divergence from what would be considered realistic. Were Irma to appear rosy-cheeked in the dream, the analysis would not have focused specifically on that content. This is, of course, not to say that Freud focuses only on the surprising or incongruent. It is not surprising, impossible, or unrealistic that Irma would be standing by a window. But here too Freud's interest in this kind of plausible event is based on the question of why a statement is being made about Irma and a window; what sense is being conveyed through the window specifically, given that in reality there occurred no meeting with her beside a window?

Thus Freud assumes that those features in the dream that are (in terms of wakeful life) surprising, unrealistic, or at least uncommon, have a meaning that is sensible and realistic. The introduction of this assumption is highly problematic because Freud sets out to *show* that his technique leads to the discovery of meaning. If at the outset he *assumes* that underlying all fragments there are sensible and realistic statements, then to a large extent he has assumed what he set out to show. It is a short step from postulating that the dream is to be translated into a series of sensible and realistic statements to an uncritical acceptance of the assumption that the dream has meaning. No grounds for this assumption are presented.[5]

The second assumption on which Freud relies is that *apparent nonsense, or contents in need of explanation, emerge from specific forms of transformation.* This assumption pertains to the kind of explanation sought when questions arise regarding the relevance or sense of the fragment. The explanations usually involve one of the following forms of transformation and combination.

a. The curious object or clause in the dream *takes the place* of what arises in association to that object: For example, Freud in his associations to "trimethylamin" asks "what was it then to which my attention was to be directed in this way by trimethylamin?" (Freud, 1900, p. 116). And he answers:

> It was to a conversation with another friend who . . . at that time confided some ideas to me on the subject of the chemistry of the sexual processes, and had mentioned among other things that he believed that one of the products of sexual metabolism was trimethylamin . . . I began to guess why the formula for trimethylamin had been so prominent in the dream . . . Trimethylamin *was* an allusion . . . to the immensely powerful factor of sexuality. (ibid., my underline)

b. The curious object or clause is a *composite* of the different objects that arise in association to it: It is possible to find in Freud's analysis of the dream a variety of subcategories of these compositions, but one can, nevertheless, speak here of a general form. This form may be seen in Freud's associations to the unusual (i.e., incongruent with reality) physical appearances of Dr. M. and of Irma. In his associations to "Dr. M. was pale, had a clean-shaven chin and walked with a limp," Freud remarks:

> That was true to the extent that his unhealthy appearance often caused his friends anxiety. The two other features could only apply to someone else. I thought of my elder brother, who is clean shaven. . . . We had had news a few days earlier that he was walking with a limp. . . . There must, I reflected, have been some reason for my fusing into one the two figures in the dream. I then remembered that I had a similar reason for being in an ill-humour with each of them. (Freud, 1900, p. 112)

And here is another example: In his associations to Irma's standing beside the window, Freud recalls another woman who had displayed a similar stance beside the window, a stance that was significant to Freud. Freud concludes: "So in the dream I had replaced my patient by her friend" (Freud, 1900, p. 110). This conclusion is in line with the form of transformation discussed above in (a). But Freud continues: "There still remained a few features that I could not attach either to Irma or to her friend: *pale, puffy, false teeth* . . . I then thought of someone else to whom these features might be alluding . . . Thus I had been confusing my patient Irma with two other people." (ibid.)

c. The curious object or clause is an attempt to *visually represent* some logical and temporal relationships: In the previous two forms of transformation we saw how various kinds of ideational and emotional ties between representations were considered to underlie and explain what makes the object or clause in the dream curious. In this category what underlies the curiousness of the object or clause is considered to be specifically the attempt to visually represent such terms as "before," "later," "because," "not," and so on. For example, it is curious to Freud that Irma is represented both as someone who is suffering because she refused his solution and as someone who is suffering because her problem is organic and as a result Freud could offer her no solutions. Freud's analysis reveals that this apparent contradiction is explained by the claim that these contradictory images represent the term "either–or." That is, the underlying sensible and realistic kind of statement must have been that she is suffering either because of one or because of another of these reasons.

In assuming that the apparently nonsensical aspects of the dream, or other of its contents that appear in need of explanation, emerge from specific forms of transformation, Freud applies a technique that goes far beyond the mere eliciting of associations to the dream. This technique involves rather the use of a set of rules of inference in relation to these associations, through which the dream's latent meaning is supposed to emerge. Once again, what we have here is a powerful assumption of what Freud had set out to find. If the technique already presumes the basic nature of the relationship between contents of the dream and their underlying meanings, then the question of whether the technique can lead to the discovery of the dream's meaning can hardly be said to be left open for an unbiased investigation. Indeed it may still be wondered whether the technique can lead to one comprehensive meaning of the dream, but the question of whether the dream contains pieces of meaningful content is obliterated. Also obliterated is the question of the nature of the processes by which the dream is obscured (the "obscuration thesis"). These are clearly assumed in the very application of the technique. Once again no justification for this consequential step is offered.

Problem 4: Theoretical associations and the neglect of qualitative differences between associations. Not all associations that arise while reflecting on the dream bear the same relationship to it. Freud disregards this fact. To illustrate the point, imagine that Freud's doorbell rings while he is in the process of associating to the image of Irma in the dream, and the thought "I wonder when I will have time to investigate my Irma dream without interruptions" passes through Freud's mind. It would seem that the status of this "association," so to speak, differs from that of how Irma resembles another woman. Although it is likely that Freud would agree that in this instance the two indeed differ, and hence that they should not be regarded as having equal or similar relevance and implications for the understanding of the dream, there are other forms of associations whose inherent distinctiveness from each other (in essence as well as in terms of relevance and implications) is by and large overlooked.

a. Associations of rules of inference: Freud, at times, mixes the theoretical inferences that he makes with more direct kinds of associations. This may be seen in some of the examples presented in the previous section. For example, the resemblance of Irma to another woman is a simple and (relatively) immediate association. In contrast, the idea that in his dream Irma *represents* this other woman, if considered to be an association, is neither simple nor immediate. Rather, it involves a conclusion based on a theoretical inference. In Freud's analysis the two kinds of associations appear side by side, and no note is made of their different status.

This is problematic for the following reason: Theoretical inferences are based on a rational understanding of the logical or conceptual relationships between one idea and another. As such, these inferences are not available to, or determined by, momentary immediate experience. To return to the example above, while Freud immediately experienced the resemblance of Irma to another woman, he did not and could not have immediately experienced the "therefore" of his proposition that *therefore* she must be representative of some attribute of this other woman. This transition is mediated by a rule of inference tying resemblance to representation. To treat these different kinds of associations as though they have the same status is to sneak in support and justification for the rule of inference by suggesting that it is as obviously valid and self-evident as the immediate experience of perception of resemblance.

Now, it may well be that Freud indeed had associations to new and special rules of inference. This would be understandable given his general interest in such rules in the context of his study of the neuroses. But this does not warrant the *application* of these rules to dream analysis. As a result of the application of these rules, the dream is shaped into meaningful contents related to the individual's life, and in the absence of justification for this application these meanings remain equally without support.

b. Associations of motives and wishes: It will be noticed that among Freud's associations to the dream, there occasionally appears the question "why." For example, Freud asks "what could the reason have been for my having exchanged her in the dream for her friend?" (Freud, 1900, p. 110). This "why" is not just another association, but rather is related to theoretical considerations. It is based on the assumption that everything that is expressed in the dream is derived from some personal motivation. Freud's preconception pertains not only to the *raising* of the question "why," but also to what may be considered a sufficient answer to this question, what may be considered an appropriate personal motivation. It is in this context that Freud's ideas on dreams as wish-fulfillments appear.

For example, Freud explains that "the words which I spoke to Irma in the dream showed that I was specially anxious not to be responsible for the pains which she still had" (Freud, 1900, pp. 108–109). And he continues, "Could it be that the purpose of the dream lay in this direction?" And later Freud asks, "What could the reason have been for my having exchanged her [Irma] in the dream for her friend?" (Freud, 1900, p. 110). And he immediately replies, "Perhaps it was that I should have *liked* to exchange her" (ibid.). Or, after seeing, by way of his associations, that he was in the dream in fact ridiculing a friend by attributing to him a nonsensical comment, Freud wonders: "But what could be my motive for treating this friend of mine so badly?" (Freud, 1900, p. 115). And once again his immediate reply: "That was a very simple matter. Dr. M. was just as little in agreement with my 'solution' as Irma herself. So . . . I revenged myself in this dream . . . on Dr. M. by the wording of the nonsensical consolation that I put into his mouth" (ibid.).

These wishes for more agreeable patients and revenge on disagreeing colleagues are illustrative of a general trend. And while they may appear to be just additional associations and immediate derivatives of the dream, these wishes, together with the appearance at specific points of the question "why" to which they are a response, are in fact founded on certain views on what motivates people. His questions of why the characters or events of the dream emerge as they do are not *immediately* sensed associatively, nor are his solutions to these questions sensed in this way. A powerful factor in determining both is his *wakeful conception* of what constitutes reasonable motivational factors.

Here again it may be the case that due to Freud's wakeful interest in wish and purpose, his free associations sometimes expressed theoretical-conceptual views. But to treat these associations as though they were telling us something real about the nature of the dream, rather than to further explore them as associations (e.g., to wonder about the significance of the fact that he thought "why"), requires further support. Alternatively, it should be acknowledged that these are not simply *free* associations but are instead associations based on powerful theoretical assumptions. For these assumptions will undoubtedly affect, not only the possibility of discovering meaning, but the very nature of the meanings that will be discovered. If, when faced with the question "Why did I dream X?," Freud will ultimately respond through an "association" that he must have wanted his dream to be that way, preferred it that way, *wished* it that way, then the conclusion that the meaning of the dream is a wish-fulfillment would be a trivial result of the method of association, not a discovery.

Problem 5: The introduction of additional arbitrary steps. This point is closely tied to the former one, in which we saw how Freud shifts from immediate associations to associations of a theoretical nature. It became apparent that what determines the shift from one to the other was the flow of Freud's associations, but not only. Also involved are questions of what makes sense and what is inexplicable in the dream. But these latter considerations were not systematically applied. Thus Freud allows himself to ask "why" at one point, while skipping this question at another point and moving on to look for additional immediate associations. Although with regard to free associations one can do nothing but accept them as they come, when it comes to theoretical considerations their application when they "come to mind" (so to speak) is problematic. There is the danger that they will come to mind only when their application will yield helpful results. It is this kind of nonsystematic application of theoretical considerations that I refer to under the heading of arbitrariness.

Another form of this arbitrariness may be seen in the *way* Freud considers his "why" questions. He seems to leave himself a large degree of freedom, at times treating them as questions referring to personal motivations (i.e., what was my motive for saying a thing like that?) and yet at other times as indications that something was transformed (i.e., since I couldn't have said a thing like that, what could what was said have represented?). For example, when Freud wonders why in his dream he attributed to Irma a pale and puffy complexion, he does not immediately turn to wonder why he would like her to have such a complexion. Rather, he turns to see what this complexion must have represented, and only after he realizes that it must have represented another woman does he turn to ask the question of what would be his motive for substituting this other woman for Irma. The danger here is that transformation will occur until personal motives are found. And there is no reason to believe a priori that the moment one hits an association that touches a possible personal motive, that that association indeed was prominent in forming the meaning of the dream. Perhaps further elaboration of the associative context is needed. Perhaps the other woman to whom Freud associated in his reflection on Irma's complexion is insignificant, and it is only because she actually represents yet some other character that she came to mind. Freud's finding a motive for her appearance curtails that possibility as well as the possibility that he would not be able to find any personal motive for the appearance of the character to whom he may have further associated.

Yet another form of arbitrariness may be seen within the transformations. As noted earlier, the fact that Irma's complexion resembles that of another woman is taken to point to the replacement of the one for the other. In the case of Dr. M., his resemblance to Freud's brother is considered indicative of the exis-

tence of a common attribute. It is important to reiterate that Freud here goes
beyond the simple provision of associations. He is not merely stating that Irma's
complexion resembles that of another woman, or that Dr. M. brings his brother
to mind. Freud, rather, is describing rules of transformation. In the first case "if
there is resemblance, then there is substitution" and in the second case "if there is
resemblance, then a common attribute is coming into play." Although the variety
and unpredictability of the associations per se do not pose any problem, a problem arises when the rules of transformation become similarly varied and unpre-
dictable. If the rules of transformation may arbitrarily change in different
contexts, then these cannot be considered to be satisfactory rules.

Further arbitrariness is to be seen more specifically in regard to the insertion of logical connections in the course of the interpretation. Here too what is
suggested is that there are rules of representation that allow for the insertion of
such connections. For example, when Freud points to the fact that his interpretation of his "specimen dream" reveals mutually exclusive explanations of the
persistence of Irma's pains, he suggests that the exclusiveness points to the
underlying presence of the connection "either–or." That is, that what is actually
expressed through the simultaneous presentation of contradictory explanations
is the presentation of alternative explanations. But on what grounds is this specific logical connection inserted? Could Freud not have concluded that what is
in fact being expressed is that he is expressing a nonsensical argument? He does
draw this latter conclusion in face of the limitations of the argument Dr. M.
puts forth in the dream, "Dysentery will supervene and the toxin will be eliminated." Another example may be seen in Freud's insertion of the causal connection. His interpretation of the dream in effect includes several causal statements
(e.g., that he wishes to harm Otto because of his too hasty adoption of a critical
stance toward him). But why the insertion of the "because" specifically at this
point? (In fact, the insertion at this point seems to stand in contradiction to
what Freud in one of his subsequent chapters presents as the formal rules guiding the insertion of logical connections. [See Freud, 1900, p. 316.]) Once again,
the large degree of freedom that Freud allows himself in such matters renders
the specific interpretation that he arrives at unexplained.

This leads us back to the wish. We have seen in the previous section how
Freud implicitly introduced a theoretical assumption regarding the wish as the
underlying meaning of the dream. By treating his associations of personal
motives and wishes as though they were telling us not only about the inner
contents of his mind, but also about the *actual* processes that influence the formation of the dream, and/or simply by not acknowledging his basic assumption of the dream's wishful meaning he made the wishful meaning suddenly
appear. The introduction of the wish in this way may also be considered a
prime and important instance of apparently arbitrary steps that Freud takes in
the course of the dream interpretation. Such steps do not lead to the conclu-

sion that the interpretative process that Freud is applying is necessary, warranted, or reasonable.

Conclusions regarding Freud's process of analysis (The First Criterion for Route C). From this analysis of Freud's procedure in his application of his technique, we must conclude that on the basis of the procedure itself and Freud's arguments in its favor there is no necessity to accept it as correct. At many points there were no self-evident reasons for his interpretative maneuvers and no reasons were offered that pointed to their validity or necessity. We noted several kinds of problems: First, the dream is fragmented in a question-begging way into fragments and then considered in terms of the ongoing meaningful events of life. Although this step is consequential in terms of the possibility of finding meaning and the kinds of meanings that could be found, no basis for it is presented. Second, Freud goes on to rely on assumptions that were supposedly unknown to him, such as the assumption that underlying the fragments of the dream are sensible and realistic statements, and the assumption of specific forms of transformation that are responsible for the apparent insensibility of the fragments. We also saw how under the guise of free associations various theoretical considerations infiltrate his interpretative steps. Most notable in this regard are the infiltration of rules of inference for determining the nature of the dream's underlying meaning; and the infiltration of the wish as the dream's actual motivational source by allowing answers to the question "why did I dream X?" to count as free associations. In addition, we took note of several apparently arbitrary steps whereby the rules that Freud implicitly applied to his dreams were not applied systematically. In an epistemological sense, we have seen that the entire process of interpretation that Freud presents is arbitrary, but this specific group of arbitrary steps differs from the others. Although the other kinds of problems point to specific directions that Freud took, to specific constraints or rules that he introduced without providing sufficient justification, here it is the absence of constraints that is noted.

All this suggests that Freud fails in his attempt to justify his technique for analyzing the meaning of the dream through Route C. According to this route, his proposed technique is to be justified step-by-step, by supplying reasons that show that each step of the process of dream interpretation is warranted. As we saw, such reasons are lacking, and the steps through which Freud attempts to take us are often arbitrary and question-begging. Thus, there is no sufficient reason to believe that Freud's maneuvers in the application of his technique are the correct ones for the discovery of meaning. Moreover, it became quite apparent that these problematic maneuvers have a marked influence on the possibility of discovering of meaning and the nature of the meaning that could be discovered.

As noted before, Freud uses two alternative routes for justifying his techniques—the one just considered here was justification through step-by-step argumentation and the other route was through showing that the technique yields interpretations that are marked by a criterion of correctness. Since the former route proved to be unsuccessful, let us now turn to examine the second.

Problems with Freud's Criterion of the Intelligibility or Coherence of the Dream Meaning (The Criterion Used for Route B). Along the second route that Freud takes in attempting to justify his dream theory he must show that his dream interpretation elicits a formal characteristic that is known to indicate that the meaning of the dream has been discovered. Here, unlike in the other route of justification discussed above, Freud does not need to explain how he came up with the technique he is using. All he needs to show is that his technique succeeds to yield the necessary sign that his interpretations are indeed correct. As far as we are concerned, he may have come up with the technique through a superstitious belief, a magic book, or some other arbitrary manner—whatever its source, the important thing is that it interprets the dream correctly, as indicated by some formal characteristic. The question is, of course, what is the nature of this formal characteristic that can show us that the interpretations produced by the technique are correct. Freud's answer is the criterion of intelligibility or coherence. He argues that the fact that the final product of the interpretive product is intelligible and coherent is proof of the fact that the true meaning was attained. In terms of the analysis of his "specimen dream," Freud's argument is that since the meaning that he arrives at through his interpretive process is one that makes the dream intelligible, since it allows all the different strange fragments of which the dream is comprised to fit together, we may conclude that the meaning is a true one and the technique is correct or valid.

As noted earlier, this criterion emerges implicitly in the course of Freud's analysis of the dream. There is no clear-cut point at which Freud shifts from the previous criterion (or route) to the present one. Rather Freud interprets fragment by fragment, as described in the previous section, and then gradually the pieces of meaning that Freud finds begin to converge. When they all fall into place along a single intentional line, Freud concludes that he has "now completed the interpretation of the dream" (Freud, 1900, p. 118). He then goes on to describe how all became intelligible through focusing on this line (p. 119).

In examining Freud's justification of his technique in the light of this criterion, I will not question the validity of the criterion *in general*, nor will I argue that Freud fails to meet the criterion. Rather I will argue that in the case of the kind of dream interpretation that Freud is doing, this criterion cannot inform us that the true meaning of the dream has been discovered. To make my point I will make use of Freud's famous puzzle analogy that he puts forth in his 1923 paper "Remarks on the theory and practice of dream-interpretation." There,

Freud speaks of the basis for the analyst's certainty at having arrived at the true meaning of the dream:

> What makes him certain in the end is precisely the complication of the problem before him, which is like the solution of a jig-saw puzzle. A coloured picture, pasted upon a thin sheet of wood and fitting exactly into a wooden frame, is cut into a large number of pieces of the most irregular and crooked shapes. If one succeeds in arranging the confused heap of fragments, each of which bears upon it an unintelligible piece of drawing, so that the picture acquires a meaning, so that there is no gap anywhere in the design and so that whole fits into the frame—if all these conditions are fulfilled, then one knows that has solved the puzzle and there is no alternative solution. (Freud, 1923, p. 116)

Here we have Freud's most explicit statement on the intelligibility criterion. Although it appeared many years after the publication of *The Interpretation of Dreams*, it would seem that its spirit pervades that earlier book.

My argument against Freud's reliance on this criterion for the justification of his technique may be seen via two major difficulties with this puzzle analogy. The first difficulty arises from the fact that it is only under certain conditions that fitting together the pieces of a puzzle can be considered to lead to its true solution. If, for example, the pieces are molded according to need, if they are extremely small pieces, if the pieces are fairly similar to each other, and so on, then fitting them together would not say much. They could have been fit together in numerous alternative ways, and there would be no way of knowing whether the true picture was attained. Freud seems to be partially aware of this and therefore speaks of irregular and crooked shaped pieces, but we must inquire whether in the case of his dream interpretation the shapes of the pieces are indeed such that this analogy is applicable. The results of such an inquiry suggest that they are not. As we have seen, the dream is fragmented into very small pieces (e.g., Irma's complexion), the fragmentation is, from an epistemological perspective, arbitrary, the meanings of the fragments are multidimensional and can potentially fit with adjacent fragments in several different ways, and so on.

There is, however, a more damaging problem with the puzzle analogy. The analogy assumes that there is a picture and there are pieces. In the context of the dream, the picture corresponds to the dream's true comprehensive meaning. To what exactly do the pieces correspond? Although Freud seems to be speaking of the fragments of the manifest dream, further thought reveals this to be a somewhat misleading proposal: the fragments of the manifest dream are not analogous to pieces of a puzzle, or fragments of a story that fall into place. Unlike a suspense murder story in which the detective puts the seemingly unrelated pieces together into a coherent plot, the Freudian dream interpreter does *not* connect pieces of the manifest dream into a coherent manifest plot. After the interpretation process, the plot of the manifest dream is just as incoherent as it was before. After all, Freud's interpretation of the dream does not change the plot of the dream (in the sense that a detective reformulates the murder plot); it only adds to it an additional underlying layer of meaning. What seems to fall together into place through the process of interpretation are not the fragments of the manifest dream itself, but rather the *meanings* that underlie the different fragments. That is, what corresponds to the puzzle piece is not, for example, Irma's unusual complexion, but what Freud concluded that that fragment represented—the other patient who was being represented through Irma's complexion. And it is the other person—not Irma's complexion—who fits together with other pieces. This implies that in Freud's analogy, what correspond to the pieces of the puzzle are not fragments of the manifest dream but rather meanings of such fragments. Each piece of the puzzle is a unit of meaning.

But if the puzzle pieces correspond to these underlying meanings, then it follows that the pieces are not *given* but rather are *created* by the awake individual when he or she comes to analyze the dream. It is up to the awake individual to determine the pieces of the puzzle—that is, the units of meanings that presumably underlie the dream. A dream interpreter is therefore analogous to a player who first shapes the puzzle pieces, in accordance with various methods between which he or she is free to choose, and only then puts them together.

Since this is the case, the puzzle analogy becomes even less relevant. When we are dealing with a picture puzzle we know that all the pieces contribute to the whole. The only question is in what way. If the pieces join together so as to form a coherent configuration, then we may assume—putting aside the problems with the shape, size, and malleability of the pieces—that it is the one that corresponds to the original puzzle, to the true picture. But suppose we were dealing with a "confused heap of fragments" of unknown origin. Or suppose we were dealing with fragments that we created in a variety of methods, and that we were free to design and redesign these fragments until they fit each other: It would then make no sense to claim that it corresponded to an original or true picture. This situation more closely resembles the one we have in the dream. We have pieces that fit together, but what does this tell us, given that we do not know in advance that these are the relevant pieces? Perhaps they fit together because we unwittingly have not taken into account many pieces that are relevant or have simply discarded those pieces that, though being relevant, could not be forced into the picture we arbitrarily created? Perhaps they fit together because we have created them with a common idea in mind such that they inevitably would fit together (e.g., that they are all related to events from everyday life or that they are all guided by some purpose)? Under such circumstances, what can the fitting together possibly tell us about anything that resembles the formation of a puzzle?

In sum, the puzzle analogy holds only as long as we are dealing with the question of whether the relevant fragments of a whole are pieced together correctly. It breaks down at the point at which we must ask whether we *have* the relevant pieces of that whole. If we do not have the right pieces, then numerous alternative explanations for their coherence arise. This is especially so when we ourselves have created all the pieces, not simply found them. The coherence may be due to our choice of pieces and the way we cut and shaped them, rather than to anything in them that has to do with solving the puzzle. This is clearly a reasonable possibility in the dream. Since Freud fails to justify the process whereby he determined the specific meanings of the dream (the first criterion), we have no good reason to believe that the pieces of meaning that we have in our hands are the ones that are appropriate for the discovery of the dream's meaning. In the absence of good reason to believe so, the intelligibility and coherence of these pieces do not tell us that we have discovered the dream's true meaning. Freud's second criterion for the justification of his technique of dream analysis is found to be inadequate and thus his second route towards this justification ultimately fails.

Conclusions Regarding Freud's Failure to Justify His Technique in His Analysis of the "Specimen Dream." We have now concluded the examination of Freud's analysis of his "specimen dream" in light of the criteria of each of the two routes for justification. The first criterion centered on the step-by-step demonstration of the correctness of the *process* of interpretation. It fails primarily because Freud introduced several constraints and rules without offering any substantial explanation (e.g., the insertion of the dream into the events of everyday life, the application of rules of transformation). The second criterion centered on the demonstration that the *result* of the process of interpretation—the final comprehensive meaning of the dream—was a correct one, independently of any argument for the appropriateness of the process of interpretation. Here the problem is that Freud's measure of correctness was the intelligibility of the overall meaning produced by the process of interpretation; and, as we have seen, this measure could not be maintained unless there was some evidence that the process used the proper fragmentation into pieces and the proper analysis of these pieces, which is to say, unless there was some evidence for the correctness of the process. But the examination of the first criterion canceled that possibility. Moreover, even if the process of interpretation could be considered justified, its nature is such (e.g., it leads to the formation of small and flexible fragments of meaning) that even then the possibility could not be ruled out that the seemingly coherent meaning is merely a result of arbitrarily putting together unrelated pieces. Ultimately, we have had to conclude that Freud's technique does not meet either of the two criteria that he seems to be using in his attempt to justify his technique. *According to his own criteria, Freud does not succeed to justify his technique.*

An Implication of Freud's Failure to Justify His Technique for His Wish-Fulfillment Thesis

Freud's failure to justify his technique in his analysis of the "specimen dream" has important implications for his claim regarding wish-fulfillment as the meaning of the dream, a claim that was to become central to the rest of Freud's argument regarding the dream, and was a very important aspect of Freud's thought on the dream in general. Freud contended that the fact that the meaning of the dream is a wish was demonstrated through the simple application of his technique to the "specimen dream." At the end of his extensive analysis of that dream he writes:

> The conclusion of the dream . . . was that I was not responsible for the persistence of Irma's pains, but that Otto was. Otto had in fact annoyed me by his remarks about Irma's incomplete cure, and the dream gave me my revenge by throwing the reproach back on to him. The dream acquitted me of the responsibility for Irma's condition by showing that it was due to other factors. . . . The dream represented a particular state of affairs as I should have wished it to be. (Freud, 1900, pp. 118–119)

He goes on to assert that "*when the work of interpretation has been completed, we perceive that a dream is the fulfilment of a wish*" (Freud, 1900, p. 121). But along with Freud's failure through his analysis of the "specimen dream" to justify his technique as a method for the discovery of meaning, there comes also his failure to show that indeed he has discovered the dream's true meaning. Hence we cannot know that the true meaning of this dream is—as Freud claimed—a wish. The present examination of Freud's analysis of the meaning of the dream draws away the most essential foundation for the claim that the nature of the meaning of the dream is a wish.

Interim Summary: The Failure of the Justification of the Technique and Implications for the Rest of Freud's Argument

Before turning to the examination of the rest of Freud's arguments in favor of his dream theory, let us take a look at the ground we have covered thus far and see how the failure of his justification of his technique influences what remains to be examined. We had begun our examination by delineating the major propositions that make up Freud's dream theory: the proposition that there is a technique that allows for the discovery of the dream's meaning (the "technique thesis"), the proposition that all dreams have meanings that in some specific way are related to the mental activity of wakeful life (the "meaning thesis"), and finally, the proposition that there are specific processes of obscuring the dream (the "obscuration thesis"). We pointed to the apparent interdependence of these propositions and to the danger that Freud's attempt at justification of his dream theory would rely on circular reasoning unless some evidence were provided that would point to the independence of his theses. We referred to this as the epistemological challenge that faces Freud. We then turned to examine Freud's actual process of justification. We noted that there were four steps to this process: the literature review, the analysis of his "specimen dream," the generalization of his finding to the claim that the meaning of the dream is a fulfillment of a wish, and then, finally, the deduction of the processes that underlie the distortion of the dream and the motives for them. Thus far we have examined the first two steps. While the first step did not contribute to the justification, we also saw that it was not an essential step. The second step, the analysis of the "specimen dream," was.

We have seen that the analysis of the "specimen dream" was an attempt to provide justification of the "technique thesis" independently of his other theses. In this attempt, Freud implicitly worked along two routes that would determine whether the technique allowed for the discovery of the meaning of the dream without having to presuppose what the nature of that meaning was (the "meaning thesis"). In this way he met the challenge that faces the "technique thesis." Freud, however, ultimately failed to justify this thesis. Along one of his routes, his criterion of step-by-step arguments showing the correctness of the procedure of the dream analysis was not met. Along the other route, his criterion of intelligibility or coherence was found to be inadequate.

We turn now to the two remaining steps of Freud's process of justification to inquire whether there Freud's theory receives the support that it needs. In these last steps we find Freud attempting to justify his "meaning" and "obscuration" theses. But what we also find is that these attempts rely heavily on the justification of the "technique thesis," on the successful analysis of the "specimen dream," and on the demonstration that the meaning of that dream is a wish. Since as we have seen it is not legitimate to rely on these foundations, Freud's arguments at this point are already severely weakened. It is also in the course of these last two steps that Freud shifts to circular reasoning. The last two justificatory steps end in total failure.

Since Freud's arguments in his remaining steps of justification are quite weak, my discussion of them will be brief and centered on the examination of a few illustrative examples. This will allow the reader to recognize the nature and limitations of Freud's thought in this context.

The Generalization of the Finding that the Meaning of the Dream Is a Fulfillment of a Wish

After the completion of his analysis of the "specimen dream" and his conclusion that it had meaning and that its meaning was a wish, Freud turns to the task of generalizing that finding. Here he attempts to justify his "meaning thesis," namely, that the proposition that all dreams have meanings that in some specific way—a wishful one—are related to the mental activity of wakeful life.

Our first concern must be to inquire whether this is a universal characteristic of dreams or whether it merely happened to be the content of the particular dream (the dream of Irma's injection) which was the first to be analyzed. For even if we are prepared to find that every dream has a meaning and a psychical value, the possibility must remain open of this meaning not being the same in every dream. Our first dream was the fulfilment of a wish; a second one might turn out to be a fulfilled fear; the content of a third might be a reflection; while a fourth might merely reproduce a memory. (Freud, 1900, p. 123)

In chapters III and IV of *The Interpretation of Dreams* Freud continues his argument by presenting his proof that the generalization from this first analysis is indeed warranted. His argument involves two steps. First, Freud points to dreams that appear on the manifest level to be a wish-fulfillments. These include (1) dreams that Freud claims can be experimentally induced, such as dreams of drinking after eating thirst-inducing anchovies right before going to sleep; (2) dreams that appear to be obvious wish-fulfillments, such as imagining oneself already up and about when one must get up, but wishes to continue sleeping. In this context Freud brings some additional dreams that he considers to be equally plain instances, such as a dream dreamt by a woman that she is having her period, the underlying wish being of not being pregnant; and (3) children's dreams, where wishes such as that of enjoying one's favorite food, longed for in the course of the day, are blatant.

The conclusion Freud would like to draw from the presentation of these dreams is that clearly dreams are often wish-fulfillments. To further support this conclusion he adduces folk wisdom. "On the whole, ordinary usage [of language] treats dreams above all as the blessed fulfillers of wishes. If ever we find our expectation surpassed by the event, we exclaim in our delight: 'I should never have imagined such a thing even in my wildest dreams'" (Freud, 1900, p. 133).

The second step in Freud's argument for generalizability of his claim regarding the wish-fulfillment meaning of the dream is to demonstrate that even in the case of dreams that appear to contradict his conclusion, an underlying wish-fulfillment nevertheless exists. Most notable among Freud's counterexamples are dreams that are immediately experienced as arousing anxiety. Freud presents the interpretation process of numerous instances of dreams that appear to be blatantly nonwish-fulfilling. The dreams arouse distress rather than satisfaction. It emerges that in these dreams the wish-fulfillment is disguised; it can find expression only in a distorted form.

This two-step argument in favor of the generalizability of Freud's wish-fulfillment claim is problematic on several accounts: First, the meaning of the "specimen dream" had been demonstrated by Freud to be a wish-fulfillment clearly in the sense of a latent wish. If it were manifest and obvious, no demonstration (and especially not the very elaborate one that Freud put forth) would be necessary. The validity of the general applicability of the thesis that dreams are wish-fulfillments would therefore have to pertain to dreams as *latent* wish-fulfillments. Presenting instances of manifest wish-fulfillment (as Freud does in the first step of this argument) would then be irrelevant.

Second, by choosing dreams with a blatant fulfillment of a wish as his starting point for the generalization of his earlier conclusion regarding wish-fulfillment—as though these blatantly wishful dream were the "simple" cases that can be investigated independently of other types of dreams—Freud biases the investigation in favor of his desired conclusion. It gives the appearance that the starting point of the study of dreams is with the recognition that there are many instances of blatant wish-fulfillment and the question we are faced with is whether it is possible to generalize from the obvious to the less obvious instances. This question is then dealt with by pointing to the processes of distortion that appear in distressing dreams and which conceal their true wish-fulfillment meaning. The obstacle in face of generalization is overcome. I contend, however, that this overcoming is illusory. The initial obstacle was not the manifest distress in certain dreams, but rather the question of whether there is justification for the claim that distortion always conceals a latent wish-fulfillment and not other latent contents or no meaningful latent contents at all. The very fact of introducing the notion of distortion then surely cannot in any way be a solution to this question. What is required is rather some evidence that indeed distortion always conceals a latent wish-fulfillment. The question is whether the various examples of dream interpretation that Freud presents provide such evidence.

The third problem with Freud's argument for the generalizability of his wish-fulfillment claim is simply that this does not seem to be the case. Even those dreams that Freud brings as examples of *manifest* wish-fulfillment are not obviously so. For these dreams to count as expressing wish-fulfillment, we would have, at the very least, to have information concerning the wishful state of the dreamer. Perhaps in the experimental thirst-induced dreams we know something of this, but we know much less regarding most of the other dreams that Freud describes. But even in such extreme experimental cases, in order to see the dream as a positive instance of wish-fulfillment we would have to know that indeed it was the *wishfulness* of the state of the dreamer that underlies the dream. Can we, for example, discard the possibility that it was the purely physical state of need that was responsible for the dream, rather than the psychical wish? If this were the case, then in line with this, someone with a vitamin C deficiency of which he has no knowledge (conscious or unconscious) may dream of drinking orange juice, although he has no *wish* in relation to either orange juice or vitamin C. To determine that the dream samples presented are indeed positive instances of wish-fulfillment requires a more careful methodological design.

Fourth, even were we to accept these examples as positive instances of manifest wish-fulfillment, they would not in themselves provide support for the *generalization* of the claim that the meaning of the dream is a wish. This would be so even were we to limit the claim to the meaning of pleasant dreams. In such a context positive instances in themselves prove little. We would have to know, for example, not only that there are pleasant dreams that can be understood in terms of the individual's state of wishfulness, but also that there are no pleasant dreams that are not. Again, a more complex design is needed. Simply bringing examples in which the hypothesis seems to have "worked" will not suffice.

These methodological difficulties are relevant also to the assessment of the value of the more complex dreams that Freud introduces, those in which the wish-fulfillment is latent. There too it cannot be concluded on the basis of the evidence provided that indeed the wish that was discovered was a wish that latently existed in the dreamer. Nor would the acceptance of such a conclusion resolve the problem (noted above) of generalization on the basis of positive instances only. But regarding these latter complex dreams there is an additional basic difficulty: Since the claim here (in contrast to the claim in relation to the manifest wish-fulfillment dreams) is that the wish-fulfillment becomes apparent only when its disguise is removed, we would have to have evidence regarding both the validity of the statement of there being a disguise, and the validity of the process by way of which it is removed. The claim that the meaning of the dream is a latent wish can only be as good and well supported as the claim that there is distortion. No new evidence in this regard is provided. Instead Freud assumes that there is distortion and relies for its removal on the same technique that he applied in his analysis of the "specimen dream," a technique that was ultimately shown to be without basis. And indeed his examples of analysis of latent wish-fulfillment dreams suffer from the same limitations and problematic maneuvers that we encountered in his interpretation of the "specimen dream."

One final problem with his generalization attempt is that it seems that now Freud uses the fact that he arrives at a wishful meaning as the sign that he has indeed correctly interpreted the dream. This is problematic because Freud, at the same time, intends to show that a wish is always the meaning of the dream by relying on the fact that this is what emerges from the correct interpretation of the dream. A vicious circularity here seeps in.

To further augment his claim regarding the general validity of the wish-fulfillment meaning of dreams, Freud employs several other arguments. I will expand here on his central argument regarding *censorship,* which is paradigmatic of his general line of thought in this context.

Freud introduces his concept of censorship in order to show the ubiquitous existence of distortive defensive motives that aim to conceal the wish-fulfillment nature of the dream. His point is as follows: One may see a similarity between censorship (both social and political) and dream distortion. In both, one's true stance is disguised. In the context of censorship the disguise is in order to express what is forbidden by the authorities. The similarity between censorship and dream distortion

> justifies us in presuming that they are similarly determined. We may there-fore suppose that dreams are given their shape in individual human beings by the operation of two psychical forces . . . and that one of these forces constructs the wish which is expressed by the dream, while the other exer-cises a censorship upon this dream-wish and, by the use of that censorship, forcibly brings about a distortion in the expression of the wish. (Freud, 1900, pp. 143–144)

It may be seen, however, that the thinking underlying this conclusion is falla-cious on two major accounts. Firstly, since—in the context of Freud's argu-ment—the fact that the dream is disguised is assumed, not discovered, the similarity between dream distortion and censorship is also assumed and not dis-covered. Hence to draw any conclusion on the basis of the similarity would be to assume it and not discover it. And if the conclusion is just a further assump-tion, the parallel is unnecessary and even misleading. It adds no evidential sup-port, but falsely appears to do so. The dream is simply construed to be similar to an expression under censorship and then the "discovery" that it is similar is presented as a source of understanding of the essential nature of the dream.

It may also be wondered here in what way Freud considered the two processes to be so very similar. He refers to them as corresponding "down to their smallest details" (Freud, 1900, p. 143). It would seem that the very fact (but actually the assumption) of there being disguised expressions is the only basis for their similarity. But such a similarity is hardly detailed. On the basis of such a similarity one would have to conclude that all disguises (e.g., costumes worn at a costume party) are based on a censorship model. There is the possibil-ity that the similarity that Freud had in mind was more specifically the interac-tion between two forces (expressive and censoring forces) that underlie the disguise in both phenomena. But if that were the case, not only would the con-clusion regarding the dream based on this similarity be no more than a further assumption regarding the dream's nature, but furthermore the conclusion would simply be tautological. Our initial assumption would be that the dream is a dis-guised expression of a wish based on the interaction between two forces, and on the basis of this assumption we would draw the conclusion that the dream is a disguised expression of a wish based on the interaction between two forces.

The second basic limitation of Freud's argument regarding dream censor-ship is that even if the parallel between dream distortion and censorship were well based and not presupposed, there is the question of whether such a parallel warrants the conclusion that the phenomena were derived from the same motives or based on the same kinds of processes. Clearly, when what is consid-ered to be similar between two phenomena is based on a very broad common denominator, (e.g., the two simply involve some kind of disguise), the conclusion that they are derived from the same motives cannot be maintained. There do not seem to be any better grounds for this conclusion when the similarity is more specific and detailed.

We may conclude here that Freud's analogy between dream distortion and censorship is far from being a well-founded argument in favor of the proposition that dream distortion aims to conceal the dream's underlying wishful nature. His analogy does not introduce new evidence or support of some other kind, but rather only additional assumptions, the basis for which has not been shown. Taken together with the problematic nature of Freud's arguments in favor of the generalization that all dreams are wishful, we may conclude that in this third step of Freud's attempt to justify his dream theory no new independent foundation for his dream theory is provided. He cannot claim to know that all dreams have meanings that are related to the psychic activity of wakeful life, nor can he, of course, claim to know the *way* in which they are related to this mental activity. Instead of a new foundation, what Freud reveals in this step are what appear to be his assumptions regarding the place of the wish and distortion in the dream, and at times a circular reasoning that emerges from his attempt to present what is assumed as a new and significant discovery.

We may now turn to the final step.

The Deduction of the Processes that Underlie the Distortion of the Dream and the Motives for Them

In introducing his concept of censorship, Freud not only attempts to buttress his argument for the general validity of the claim that dreams are wish-fulfillments, but also moves on to the elaboration of his ideas on the processes that underlie the distortion of the dream. Here we have Freud's "obscuration thesis." In this context the major issue is the nature of the dream work. That is, what kinds of processing are responsible for the transformation of the dream thoughts (the meanings) that underlie the dream into what appears in the dream content, in the manifest dream?

The Nature of the Dream Work

Freud's ideas on the dream work are elaborated in the course of his long and complex chapter VI. His aim is to describe the processes responsible for the transformation of the thoughts underlying the dream into the dream itself, that is, into the manifest dream content. He intends to do this by way of deduction. He writes:

> The dream-thoughts and the dream-content are presented to us like two versions of the same subject-matter in two different languages. Or more properly, the dream-content seems like a transcript of the dream-thoughts into another mode of expression, whose characters and syntactic laws it is our business to discover by comparing the original and the translation. (Freud, 1900, p. 277)

Here too, however, one must ultimately conclude that Freud does not make a new discovery but rather merely reiterates earlier assumptions. What we have here is not a process of deduction, as his translation analogy would lead one to believe, but rather an inverted reading of what Freud had already assumed when he applied his technique to the discovery of the meaning of the dream. In our discussion of the challenge that Freud faces in his attempt to justify his "obscuration thesis," it was this problem that had to be overcome. Freud did not overcome it. Let us see why.

Freud in this context is not "*presented*" with two versions of the dream, as he claims. He is presented with one alone—that of the manifest dream, the "dream-content version." The second version, that of the dream thoughts, is one that he, Freud, produces himself. It is only through the application of his method that this second version is determined. Once this is recognized, it becomes clear that the dream work is, and can be nothing but, the various rules that Freud devised and used as he applied his technique of dream interpretation, now in reverse.

Freud does not recognize this and goes into great detail regarding the deduction of the various dream-work processes. He explains, for example, how one comes to know of condensation, the process whereby two or more underlying ideas or images find expression in a single manifest content. Freud claims that it becomes necessary to assume condensation when one recognizes how brief the dream is in comparison to the vast amount of associations it generates—all of which are, according to him, related to the underlying dream thoughts. Analysis of the actual process that led Freud to this conclusion, however, puts it in question. It may be seen that the idea that all the associations to the dream thoughts are related to the underlying dream thoughts is based on Freud's method, or rather on an assumption within his method. Freud had sought associations to the various parts of the dream, and he assumed these to be relevant and related to the underlying meaning of these parts. Clearly, asking for associations to a specific part will ultimately generate more associations than parts and if one assumes these to be related, then basically condensation is being assumed. Condensation is not discovered; rather it is inherent to an assumption regarding the technique.

Another example may be seen in the way Freud claims to have discovered displacement, the process by which remote elements take the place of psychically charged ones. He shows how he deduced the influence of this process from the numerous dream interpretations he has carried out. He presents the reader with quite a few examples of these in order to demonstrate his point: For example, "In my dream about my uncle, the fair beard which formed its centre-point seems to have no connection in its meaning with my ambitious wishes which as we saw were the core of the dream-thoughts. . . . Dreams such as these give a justifiable impression of 'displacement'" (Freud, 1900, pp. 305–306). Ostensibly, it is the comparison of the manifest dream with the latent dream thoughts that leads to the discovery of the process. But here too, an analysis of the actual course of events reveals that were it not for the fact that Freud knew of the process of displacement and assumed it as part and parcel of his technique, he would not have been able to discover it. Freud *assumed* that it was a significant fact that in his dream he portrayed his friend with the yellow beard of his uncle; that indeed it indicated that he equated his black-bearded friend R. with his fair-bearded uncle, with all the ambition-related aspects of the equation. It was on the basis of this assumption that he concluded that there were two texts— the manifest one having to do with his friend strangely having a fair beard, and the latent one having to do with his ambitions. What can emerge from the comparison of the two texts is thus heavily determined by the assumptions that were used in their discovery in the first place. The texts were not presented to Freud independently of his technique. (The reader may take note that here Freud relies on the first rule of transformation that we discussed in the context of the problems with the justification of his technique.) Freud thus discovers (now in reverse) what he had originally assumed.

The presentation of the dream-work processes as discoveries deduced from the comparison of two texts related to the dream continues throughout. It becomes most blatant in Freud's discussion of "means of representation," the means by which various kinds of connections between ideas—such as those of causation, alternative, contradiction, similarity, and so on—can be represented in the dream. The claim that "simultaneity in time" points to a logical connection, that certain forms of transformations of objects or images in dreams or their sequential appearance point to a causal relation, that unification of objects or images points to their underlying similarity, and so on—all these are implicitly assumed in the course of applying the technique to produce the alleged meaning of the manifest dream. Hence they cannot be later presented as something simply deduced from a comparison of the manifest and the latent texts. We had discussed these rules of transformation and Freud's assumption of them in the context of the problems with his justification of his technique. We had, for example, seen how Freud's rule that "unification of images indicates their similarity" was assumed in his analysis of his "specimen dream." There Freud considered the fact that Irma's image in the dream contained attributes that did not in reality belong to her to indicate that some kind of similarity exists between Irma and other people with whom Freud did associate these attributes.

Beyond any specific example, however, the point is that unless there is some independence between the process of transforming the manifest text of the dream into the latent dream-thought version (i.e., the technique of dream interpretation) and the process by which the latent dream thought version is transformed into the manifest dream (i.e., the dream work), it is not possible to speak of the *discovery* of the relationship between the two, or of the *discovery* of the nature of the processing that takes place between them. If the second text emerges through the application of a completely established technique of "decodification" of the first text, then it is not legitimate to suggest that the comparison of the texts will *reveal* "the characters and syntactic laws" of this first text (Freud, 1900, p. 277). For all these were already assumed and used when the first text was translated into the second. For it to be otherwise, the process of transformation of the second text into the first would have to have some independence from the process of transformation of the first into the second. There would then be two texts and the questions would be: In what ways are they related? What kinds of processes must underlie the transformation of the one into the other? This, however, is not the situation in the case of the process of transformation that Freud offers us.

Brief Conclusion Regarding the Value of Freud's Last Two Steps in His Process of Justification

The present examination of Freud's third and fourth steps in his process of justification point to the fact that they do not provide a new foundation for Freud's dream theory. Freud's contention that all dreams have certain kinds of meaning (i.e., wishful ones) that are related to the ongoing psychic activity of wakeful life here appears to rely on the validity of his technique, on the success of analysis of his "specimen dream," on the discovery of the wishful meaning of that dream, and on faulty arguments in favor of generalizing the latter finding. And his contentions regarding the nature of the obscuring processes and the motives underlying them were revealed to be the result not of the deductive process which Freud claimed to have done, but rather were already embedded in Freud's technique. By relying on support of this kind, a new foundation cannot be secured. Rather, relying on this support places the dream theory within a web of circular reasoning. In these last steps, Freud merely finds what he has already assumed. Nothing new is contributed. The last two steps of justification are of no value whatsoever to Freud's epistemological project.

AN OVERVIEW OF FREUD'S EPISTEMOLOGICAL PROJECT

The Nature of Freud's Epistemological Project: Meaning, Truth, and Justification

In contrast to the critical studies of Freud's dream theory offered by Grünbaum and Spence, the present study followed Freud's path, step-by-step, as he presented and attempted to justify his theory. This detailed investigation of Freud's reasoning enables us now to assess more accurately the nature of Freud's epistemological project, especially with respect to the basic concepts discussed in chapter 1, such as those of meaning and truth. This allows not only for a more accurate understanding of the nature of the dream theory that Freud wished to justify and the reasons why his justification failed, but also for determining alternative possibilities of justification. Different kinds of propositions may require, or be amenable to, different kinds of justification, and the presence of obstacles impeding justification is determined by the kind of justification that was attempted. Before we proceed, let us therefore take stock of what can now be seen concerning the nature of Freud's project.

Meaning as "Meaning Discovered"

First, it should now be clear that Freud aims at what I called "meaning discovered," and not at all at "meaning described" or "meaning created." Specifically, in the course of our examination we have seen how Freud's concern is with discovering the meaning of the dream in the sense of discovering the actual connections within the mind that underlie the dream. This is apparent throughout his arguments and most directly in his delineation of the three propositions that he intends to justify. There, for example, he speaks of revealing the dream as a meaningful psychical structure. Such a structure is clearly not a created entity that could have been different depending on the way the analyzers connect the themes. This structure rather refers to something that actually exists in the individual's mind. Here we also see Freud's realism with respect to psychic states. Meanings exist; they are psychic structures in the mind, and the question is whether we can reveal them, bring them to light.

The Correspondence Theory of Truth

This leads us to Freud's conception of the notion of truth. As Freud presents his propositions concerning these meanings, his reliance on a correspondence theory of truth is apparent. The truth of interpretations of specific dreams, or of broader theoretical propositions regarding the nature of dreams is determined by whether it corresponds to the facts. The interpretations and propositions must fit the dream material, which stands as an extra-theoretical datum. That is, Freud would not consider the dream material to be just another theoretical proposition that is subject to change just like any other, and whose truth depends on whether or not it fits into the coherent set of propositions. For Freud the objective empirical data express the hard facts that a theory must correctly explain in order to be true.

Meaning of Stating and Meaning of the Statement

The truth with which Freud is primarily concerned is that all dreams have meanings that are accessible through the application of the psychoanalytic technique. This is the essence of Freud's dream theory. The three propositions—the "technique thesis," the "meaning thesis," and the "obscuration thesis"—all ultimately point to Freud's concern with the possibility of uncovering meanings in the dream through the application of the psychoanalytic technique and the application of basic psychoanalytic rules of transformation (e.g., displacement). We also saw, however, how in the course of the work—after his analysis of the "specimen dream"—Freud shifted from the aim of showing that dreams have meaning to showing that the dreams have meaning of a specific kind, namely, a wishful kind. In other words, the emphasis in the "meaning thesis" (i.e., that all dreams have meanings that in some specific way are related to the mental activity of wakeful life) now seems to have moved from the very meaningfulness of all dreams to the fact of the meaningfulness being of a specific kind.

One may regard Freud's emphasis on the specific wishful nature of the dream as merely a further elaboration of the proposition that the dream is meaningful. Not only is the dream meaningful, but its meaning is always of a certain kind. The analysis in the previous chapter of the notion of meaning suggests, however, a more radical understanding of the status of the wishfulness hypothesis, one that has not yet been observed in the literature. In that chapter, I made a distinction between two types of meaning that Freud was interested in discovering: the meaning of the statement (what is meant or expressed through the statement, e.g., through a dream) and the meaning of stating (why the statement, e.g., a dream, was made; what psychic forces motivated its expression). For Freud, both were central aspects of the meaning of a given expression. Now, when Freud speaks of the meaning of the dream he is referring both to the underlying unconscious intentions that find expression in the dream (e.g., "I really did mean that my friend R. was a simpleton—like my Uncle Josef" [p. 139]), and to the psychic forces that motivated the dream (e.g., Freud's wish to receive the title of professor). I suggest that these two can be seen as reflecting the distinction between the two types of meaning. The proposition that the dream is meaningful and the proposition that the meaning of the dream is a wish, may be considered to refer to the meaning of the statement and the meaning of stating respectively. In other words, when Freud proposes that all dreams have meaning, he is claiming that all dreams express latent connections between psychic entities (e.g., between Freud's idea of his friend R. and his idea of his uncle Josef). And when Freud proposes that the meanings of all dreams are wishes, he is claiming that all dreams are motivated by a wish (e.g., Freud expressed the connection between R. and Josef because he had a wish to state that R. was a simpleton, as part of a broader wish of Freud's to receive the title of professor). It follows that the wish is not an inherent part of the statement per se, but rather of the motivating force for its expression. The nature of the statement is unlimited. It is only when one turns to the question of why someone would be making such a statement that the limiting factor of the wish is introduced. This wish can only be seen in the light of the individual's broader wakeful personality. It does not reside within the statement itself. For example, in Freud's analysis of his "specimen" he ultimately comes to the conclusion that it means that he is not responsible for Irma's illness. The statement that he is not responsible for Irma's illness is, however, not in itself a wish. It is only in the light of Freud's fear that he was being accused of this that the exoneration is wishful. Were Freud to have strong sado-masochistic tendencies, it may be difficult to consider this statement to be an expression of a wish.

One consequence of this understanding of the relationship of Freud's proposition regarding meaning in the dream in general to his proposition regarding the wishful meaning of the dream is that the latter can be discarded without denying the significance of the former. It is true that Freud's expectation that the motive of the dream is a wish (i.e., that this is the meaning of stating it) influences his interpretation of what the dream says (i.e., the meaning of the statement). (This influence takes place, e.g., through the way Freud introduces in his associations the question "why.") Nevertheless, it is in principle possible to relate to Freud's more basic and central proposition that dreams have psychoanalytically discoverable meaning while neglecting his proposition regarding the wish.

Forms of Justification

The basic and central proposition that dreams have meanings (in the sense of meaning of the statement) that are accessible through the psychoanalytic technique is also the subject of the more serious attempt at justification than his proposition concerning the wishfulness of the dream. A few sections ago, we saw that that latter proposition relies heavily on the proof that the first one is true, and that it suffers from circular and convoluted reasoning. It became clear that it is far from obvious that the "simple" dreams indeed express wishful thinking, that their choice as a starting point did not distort the picture, and that the generalization from these special cases to all dreams was justified. In contrast, we saw earlier in the chapter that Freud devotes a much more comprehensive and well-thought through attempt to justify his claim about the very meaningfulness of the dream. Here Freud relies on two criteria: the demonstration that each step in the long process of the dream analysis is warranted, and the intelligibility or coherence of the interpretation produced by the technique.

We may now view these criteria in the light of the broad map of possible forms of justification that was set forth in chapter 1. When Freud comes to justify his dream theory he always maintains that the empirical data should serve as the foundation for his theoretical formulations. These theoretical formulations form a superstructure built on the empirical foundations, in this case the data of the dreams themselves, and they will be justified only when they account for this data. As he later explains in one of his most direct statements on his view of the scientific status of psychoanalysis: "Ideas are not the foundation of science, upon which everything rests: that foundation is observation alone. They are not the bottom but the top of the whole structure" (Freud, 1914, p. 77). Accordingly, nowhere in the course of his extended process of justification do we find Freud willing to dispense with his observed dream data. Rather, he works incessantly to show that his interpretations and theoretical propositions can account for it. In contrast to coherentist approaches to justification, Freud does not put the data itself in question or consider discarding or modifying parts of it in order to enhance the coherence of his theoretical propositions.

Freud adopts two forms of a Foundationalist approach, one form completely Atomistic and the other containing a minimal degree of Holism. His Atomism is most marked when he relies on the first criterion, that of demonstrating the step-by-step correctness of his technique of interpreting dreams. As he puts forth his long series of arguments in favor of each of the steps he takes in the course of his interpretation of the "specimen dream," Freud is attempting to support his proposition that the meaning of the dream can be discovered through the application of his technique in isolation from any other psychoanalytical proposition. His arguments attempt to show that this specific proposition, independently of the psychoanalytic theory as it applies to other domains, allows for the correct analysis of the data (i.e., the interpretation of the manifest dream). In Freud's second criterion for justification, we see a slightly more Holistic approach. Freud's reliance on intelligibility or coherence as indicating that the true meaning of the dream has been reached points to his adoption of coherence as a criterion for justification. It is the way in which all the pieces of the dream come together into the single comprehensive meaning that (purportedly) justifies his proposition that he has indeed discovered the dream's true meaning. This is a holistic element of justification because it is the fitting together of different pieces of data that makes the interpretation justified.

In this context it is very important to take note of two points. First, the fact that Freud uses coherence as a criterion for justification does not in any way mean that he has adopted a Coherence theory of justification. As we saw in chapter 1, not only Coherence theory but also Holistic Foundationalism uses coherence as a criterion of justification. The difference is that the former takes coherence to be the sole criterion of justification without any special regard for the data, while the latter may use coherence—and/or other criteria—in the attempt to form a body of theoretical of propositions that will be justified to the extent that they account for the data. And indeed, the data for Freud still maintain a special status, and he seeks to justify his theoretical propositions on their basis. Second, the Holism that Freud seems at times to be using is of a very minimal kind. This is Holism within the body of data related to a given dream, but the theoretical proposition, the interpretation in this case, is still determined without reference to any broader framework. Here too Freud does not rely on the broader network of psychoanalytic propositions in his process of justification. The specific proposition is seen as standing on its own and is tested accordingly. In fact, the Holism is so minimal in this case that it may be regarded as primarily Atomistic.

I have thus far focused on the most significant of Freud's propositions, namely, that the dream has accessible meaning. In this context we have found his process of justification to be based on a mainly Atomistic Foundationalist approach. As noted earlier, Freud's other proposition concerning the wishful meaning of the dream is based on the justification of the first proposition as well as on additional circular and convoluted reasoning. There too, however, we find that Freud continues to regard the data with special reverence and to focus on the justification of his propositions in isolation from the broader theoretical framework of psychoanalysis. Freud attempts to account for the data through single propositions, rather than through networks of related propositions. Thus we may conclude that the nature of Freud's process of justification in regard to his dream theory is essentially Atomistic Foundationalist.

We may now turn to discuss the failure of this method of justification of Freud's dream theory.

The Failure of Freud's Epistemological Project

The Fact of Failure

Since a large part of this chapter has been devoted to the description of the multiple ways in which Freud's process of justification has failed, I will here only briefly summarize the conclusions. Let us begin with the very fact that Freud did not succeed to justify his theory of dreams. From the outset we saw that given the nature of Freud's theses—the "meaning thesis," the "technique thesis," and the "obscuration thesis"—there were important challenges that would have to be overcome in order to justify his theory. His theses appeared to be mutually interdependent and were he not to find for them some independent support, they would be based on circular reasoning. For example, in the absence of independent support there was the danger that Freud's technique would be justified by its success in arriving at the correct meaning of the dream, and the correctness of the meaning would be determined by the fact that it was discovered through the application of the correct technique.

The present study shows that it is, in fact, only regarding the "technique thesis"—the thesis that there is a technique that allows for the discovery of the dream's meaning—that Freud succeeds in delineating a way for justification that can overcome the challenges. Only here does he propose criteria for justification that do not rely on, or assume, the other two theses. In the other two theses Freud found himself caught in a web of interrelated ideas without any new and independent basis for their justification. This was most blatant regarding the "obscuration thesis" in which Freud merely found what he had assumed in the application of his technique.

Although Freud delineated two independent criteria for noncircular justification of the "technique thesis"—a step-by-step proof of the technique's correctness and the intelligibility or coherence of its products—we saw that ultimately he failed to show that his technique succeeds in terms of either of the two. On the first, step-by-step proof, Freud failed because his arguments were not convincing. He made many interpretative maneuvers, maneuvers that clearly determined the possibility of discovering meaning and the nature of the meaning that could be discovered, without providing adequate reasons. Why insert the dream into the context of the events of everyday life? Why fragment the dream in this way rather than another? Why assume that underlying the fragments of the dream are sensible and realistic statements, or that there are specific forms of transformation that are responsible for the apparent insensibility of the fragments? and so on. There is simply not sufficient reason to believe that the maneuvers that Freud takes in the application of his technique are the correct ones for the discovery of meaning.

Concerning Freud's second criterion, we recognized its dependence on the first. The coherence that Freud sought was not between given pieces of the dream, but between pieces of meaning, ones that he himself had created. If their creation was not legitimate, then the coherence between them may not be telling us anything regarding the meaning of the dream. Moreover, the kinds of pieces of data between which Freud was seeking coherence were such that it was possible that they could cohere in a variety of ways, many of which would have nothing to do with the dream's meaning. Coherence is not a magic formula for solving all problems in all cases.

Since Freud's other two basic theses—his "meaning thesis" and his "obscuration thesis"—do not rely on additional new evidence or new forms of arguments, we had to conclude that they too do not offer any new foundation for Freud's dream theory. Ultimately we had to conclude that Freud's justification of his dream theory failed.

A Broader Look at the Reasons for the Failure: The Latent Influence of the Psychoanalytic Framework

We may now take a step back and put aside the numerous details of the failure of Freud's Atomistic attempt of justification of his dream theory and turn to the question of whether there is something in Freud's general strategy that was responsible for the failure. Can we discern some broad problem with Freud's approach that underlies this failure? In the course of our examination we noted two basic problems in this regard. The first problem is that Freud seems to be working within the framework of numerous constraints, assumptions, and rules without explicitly acknowledging doing so (e.g., the insertion of the dream into the events of everyday life, the application of rules of transformation). Within the context of Freud's Atomistic justification, these unacknowledged assumptions, constraints, and rules are merely arbitrary procedures that render the steps that Freud is taking unnecessary and inexplicable. After all, Atomism means that each specific issue is treated in its own terms, and that it is impossible to import ideas from other domains.

The second and related problem is the fact that Freud's data are not simply given to him. The facts with which the theoretical propositions are to correspond are not immediately available. The manifest dream itself may be considered an immediate observation, but this was not the data that Freud was actually working with. As we saw in our study of Freud's second implicit criterion in his justification of the "technique thesis" (the criterion of the coherence produced by the final product of the interpretation), the data are the pieces of meaning *underlying* the manifest dream. Freud creates his data; he does not find it. Unless we have good reason to believe that it is legitimate to create the data in the way that he did, we cannot consider the coherent interpretation that it produces to be indicative of the dream's true meaning.

To these two basic problems we should add Freud's ongoing problems with circularity, and with presenting discoveries that on further inspection emerge as mere elaborations of his own assumptions.

Looking at the nature of the broad problems that underlie the failure of Freud's Atomistic justification process, we may conclude that the major obstacle to success appears to be the fact that when he tested his theses in isolation from the rest of his psychoanalytic theory he maintained various preconceptions regarding the nature of meaning, the ways in which underlying meaning find expression and are transformed, the pervasive role of the wish in psychic life, and so on, that he did not neutralize when he set out to test his dream propositions.

But where are these preconceptions from? Are they indeed arbitrary? The answers to these questions lead us to the essential reason for the collapse of Freud's epistemological project. Looking at the detailed list of problems with Freud's justification, we may see that most of the unacknowledged constraints, the arbitrary moves, the inexplicable rules, can in fact be tied to basic psychoanalytic conceptions that Freud had already applied in his work with neurotics. Freud had maintained that neurotic symptoms should be seen in the context of meaningful events of everyday life, that they are meaningful statements, that to determine their meanings one must trace them back to their meaningful origin by way of certain methods of transformation, and so on. (Breuer & Freud, 1895). Also, in his work on neurosis Freud was developing a conception of human behavior according to which its basic motivational factor was the wish, the search for pleasure (Freud, 1950 [1895]). This is a very significant point in the understanding of the failure of Freud's attempt at justification. *Freud's process of dream interpretation was embedded within a theoretical system that Freud assumed but did not bring to the fore.* He did not put it on the table. And yet he did not ignore it. Although he tested his theses in isolation from the rest of his psychoanalytic theory, he did not appropriately silence ideas that originated in this larger theoretical context. His theoretical preconceptions were infiltrating and guiding him throughout the analysis of his dreams. The result was the emergence of apparently arbitrary and circular maneuvers and discoveries of what Freud seemed to have already assumed. In sum, Freud's failure was really a failure of the Atomistic justification of the dream theory.

Implications for the Possibility of Justification of Freud's Dream Theory

Faced with Freud's failure to justify his dream theory, primarily his proposition that the meaning of the dream is accessible through the application of the psychoanalytic technique, there are several possible positions that one could assume regarding the potential value of that theory. Although there is no room for Spence's call for the application of more rigorous criteria for justification—Freud's are sufficiently rigorous—one may adopt Grünbaum's position that Freud's theory is unfounded, or his more extreme position that the theory is simply wrong. This would imply abandoning the clinical practice of dream interpretation. Alternately, one could adopt a psychoanalytical hermeneuticist approach. Accordingly, one would continue with dream interpretation, while assuming that the meanings that are derived from the process have nothing to do with actual connections between psychic entities that are expressed through the dream. Both of these positions imply abandoning the possibility that the psychoanalytic technique could lead us to the discovery of the true meaning of the dream.

I suggest that there is a third position that leaves room for this possibility. *This third position is to explore the possibility of a Holistic Foundationalist justification for the dream theory.* Freud's justification fell through because he worked within a theoretical network while adopting an Atomistic approach to justification. Were Freud to acknowledge the inherent embeddedness of his dream theory, matters would have been different. Were Freud to recognize that he is using a network of propositions that rely on each other to account for the empirical evidence, then instead of trying to show that a single proposition regarding the dream can provide an account of the evidence, he would try to support the proposition within a broader context. He could then try to show that this proposition fits well into the overall network of ideas with which he is working, and that taken together with the other propositions of the network it provides a broader framework that is well founded on the evidence and explains it adequately.

Freud did not acknowledge the inherent embeddedness of his dream theory within the broader psychoanalytic frame and did not offer a Holistic Foundationalist justification. Perhaps in the early years of psychoanalysis in which Freud was developing his dream theory it would have been presumptuous to attempt to justify his theory by relying on the broader psychoanalytic framework. The broader framework itself was not yet considered a sufficiently acceptable model for the dream theory to rely on it. Another explanation of the absence of Holistic justification in Freud's writing is the fact that at the beginning of the twentieth century this form of justification had not yet been clearly spelled out, although in practice science has always adopted a Holistic approach. And yet, the way that Freud went about interpreting dreams, the way in which his dream theory was embedded within the broader psychoanalytic framework, cries out for a Holistic justification. Rather than denigrate the theory and discard it as Grünbaum suggests, rather than denigrate the theory and adopt it as suggested by the hermeneuticists, there is the possibility of responding to this cry. The time has come to examine whether the dream theory may be justified Holistically.

As a matter of fact, there are points at which his Holism not only lies latently in the background of his Dream Book, but rather finds more direct and formal expression. For example, towards the end of *The Interpretation of Dreams* Freud writes:

> No conclusions upon the construction and working methods of the mental instrument can be arrived at or at least fully proved from even the most painstaking investigation of dreams or of any other mental function taken in *isolation*. To achieve this result, it will be necessary to correlate all the established implications derived from a comparative study of a whole series of such functions. (Freud, 1900, p. 511)

This formal view does not, however, find expression when Freud actually comes to justify his dream theory. One may perhaps argue that Freud's statement that the technique that he is applying to the dream was the one he applied to the understanding of neurotic symptomology suggests that in practice Freud applies a Holistic form of justification. According to this view, when Freud states that "It was then only a short step to treating the dream itself as a symptom and to applying to dreams the technique of interpretation that had been worked out for symptoms" (Freud, 1900, p. 101), he is in fact justifying the application of the technique to the dream through the relationship that exists between his propositions regarding the dream and neuroses. But, as we saw in our earlier

discussion of this remark, Freud offers no explanation of the nature of the relationship between the two. He does not set forth any arguments as to why it
would be legitimate to apply to the dream a technique that was applied to neurotic symptoms. Consequently, we had to conclude that this statement regarding the application of the technique was a descriptive statement rather than an
attempt at justification. That is, the statement merely describes how Freud came
across the technique, but does not tell us anything regarding why its application
to the dream is justified.

To Holistically justify the thesis that the psychoanalytic technique can
lead to the discovery of the meanings of dreams, it is not enough to simply
insert the dream into the broader psychoanalytic framework as Freud did. It is
not enough to assume, as Freud did, that the technique that he applied in his
work with neurotic symptoms is appropriate to the dream, that like in the case
of such symptoms dreams belong to the context of meaning of everyday life,
that their underlying meanings find expression according to certain rules of
transformation, and so on. What is necessary is to show that the insertion of the
dream into the psychoanalytic framework is a legitimate maneuver.

In the next chapter I will explore the possibility of Holistically justifying
the psychoanalytic theory of dreams. There the central question will be whether
indeed it is legitimate to consider the dream a kind of context to which the network of psychoanalytic propositions regarding the discovery of meaning in general may apply. If it is legitimate, then we will have uncovered a foundation for
the psychoanalytic theory of dreams. If it is not, we will have to conclude that
we cannot know whether the application of the psychoanalytic method to the
dream allows for the discovery of the dream's meaning. As we will see, it is a
very difficult task to secure the required foundation.

After recognizing, in chapter 3, some of the obstacles to a Holistic justification of the dream theory, we will turn to see whether theoretical developments since 1900 in the areas of meaning and justification can remove these
obstacles. Although Freud's most comprehensive statement on dream theory
and its justification is expressed in *The Interpretation of Dreams*—and he always
kept that book up to date with his later thought—it is important to examine
whether any of his later, more fragmented statements in this regard shed light
on the possibility of justification. Similarly, it is important to see whether other
analysts have made contributions that resolve the difficulties that stand in the
way of justification. This exploration will provide a basis for understanding the
nature and uniqueness of the solution to the difficulties that I will set forth in
chapter 5.

CHAPTER THREE

Can the Application of Psychoanalytic Principles to the Dream be Justified?

> Yea, so far prevails the illusion of the image, in my soul and in my flesh, that, when asleep, false visions persuade to that which when waking the true cannot. Am I not then myself, O Lord my God? And yet there is so much difference betwixt myself and myself, within that moment wherein I pass from waking to sleeping, or return from sleeping to waking!
>
> —St. Augustine, *The Confessions of St. Augustine*

We turn now to the exposition and critical study of a Holistic Foundationalist form of justification of the psychoanalytic dream theory. Here the focus is on the question of whether the way in which Freud implicitly considered the dream theory as part of the broader psychoanalytic theory is a legitimate one. More specifically, the question to be examined is: *Is it legitimate to apply to the dream the general psychoanalytic principles and technique by way of which meaning is discovered?*

In addressing this question my strategy will be: (1) to first specify the assumptions on which psychoanalysis's general theory of meaning-discovery rests, (2) to examine the kind of evidence upon which these assumptions rest, and then (3) to examine whether equivalent evidence for these assumptions is available in the context of the dream.

If this kind of evidence does exist, then the application of psychoanalysis's general assumptions regarding the discovery of meaning may be legitimately applied to the dream. We may then conclude that the psychoanalytic dream theory is justified, in the sense of its being just as well founded as the psychoanalytic theory in general. In other words, psychoanalysis has certain basic assumptions regarding wakeful productions and the state of the individual producing them that lie at the foundation of its general claim that their meanings may be discovered through the application of the psychoanalytic method. If there is evidence that makes it reasonable to apply the very same assumptions to the context of the dream, then the application of the psychoanalytic method to the discovery of the dream's meaning is just as justified as the application of that method to the discovery of the meaning of wakeful products. It would then be legitimate to insert the dream into the broader psychoanalytic framework.

If, however, no such evidence is available, then these general psychoanalytic assumptions could not be applied and the claim that meaning is discovered through the application of the psychoanalytic method to the context of the dream would be unjustified.

As we will see, there is indeed an obstacle to the immediate acceptance of the general assumptions when it comes to the dream. For the psychoanalytic dream theory to be justified in a Holistic way this obstacle must be overcome.

ASSUMPTIONS UNDERLYING THE GENERAL PSYCHOANALYTIC THEORY OF DISCOVERY OF MEANING

What exactly the psychoanalytic method of discovering meaning is and what the underlying processes through which it operates are, are broad and controversial issues. Different subtheories within psychoanalysis differ on this crucial point. Many dimensions are involved in the formulation of the method and the related processes, such as the analytic relationship, interpretation, reality, and fantasy. And the nature and significance of these dimensions have been portrayed in a variety of ways (Blass & Blatt, 1992). Here my objective is not to encompass this huge complex issue. Rather, my objective is to take a meta-theoretical perspective that will allow us to stand above theoretical differences and observe what is essential to any psychoanalytic conception of discovering meaning (in the sense of "meaning discovered"). *My objective is to formulate the assumptions underlying the method of free association and of attunement to the connections between the associations that are necessary for that method to indeed allow for discovery of personal latent meanings.* My approach is minimalistic. That is, will be clear that if one wishes to further elaborate various aspects of the psychoanalytic method (e.g., to include the role of relationship), then further assumptions will be required. For our purposes the three assumptions that I will put forth here suffice.

Further Analysis of "Meaning Discovered":
A Model for the Understanding of the Assumptions

In chapter 1 we discussed the concept of "meaning discovered." At this point it is important to return to that discussion and from there further elaborate and analyze the concept. This will provide a more in-depth working model of the internal states and processes underlying the discovery of meaning, which is necessary to understand the assumptions that underlie the general psychoanalytic theory of discovering meaning.

In developing this model I focus only on those dimensions that are significant to the present study, and thus my discussion should in no way be understood as a proposal of a comprehensive and detailed model of meaning. What I am aiming for is a clear and basic statement that will explain what the discovery of meaning means in psychoanalysis, in a way that overcomes some of the difficulties of traditional formulations and some of the obscurities of more clinically oriented contemporary ones. That is, the common notions of making the unconscious conscious, or of bringing the id under the control of the ego, do not fully capture the discovery of meaning as we have come to recognize it through the many decades of psychoanalytic practice. Nor do the clinically oriented notions of the integration of meaning into the self truly formulate and explain what it is exactly that transpires in the process of discovery. Although my focus will be on making a clear and basic statement that will allow for a presentation of the assumptions underlying psychoanalysis's method of discovering meaning, it may, however, become apparent that the model of meaning that I put forth—precisely because of its very basic nature—has implications for the understanding of a range of psychoanalytical issues. It sheds light on the concepts of self, self-integration, self-development, and the nature of the relationship of these to Freud's structural model. The discussion of these concepts is, however, beyond the scope and aim of the present work and deserves extensive attention in their own right elsewhere.

In chapter 1, in our discussion of the "meaning of the statement," I had posited that meaning refers to a relationship between two entities and that in psychoanalysis, in contrast to other disciplines, this relationship is between two psychic events or states of having contents. To use the example mentioned earlier, a satisfactory psychoanalytic understanding of the meaning of "happiness" would refer to other psychic states, such as having the feeling of being admired by a significant person, or the idea of having fulfilled an Oedipal wish. I then went on to describe three broad categories of meaning, each corresponding to a form of *relationship* between psychic events. "Meaning described" referred to an experiential relationship, "meaning created" to a thematic relationship, and "meaning discovered" to a causal relationship. Ultimately, I pointed to how Freud's concern in relation to the dream was with the latter.

In that earlier discussion, the category of "meaning discovered" was defined by causation in a broad-reaching, encompassing way. What I had stated was: That when we say that X means Y, we mean that in some way Y brought about the appearance of X or influenced the way in which it appeared. This connection does not have to be experienced, nor does there necessarily have to be a thematic tie between the two (although in psychoanalysis there usually is). In our example of "happiness" this would mean that the state of happiness and the state of admiration would be *causally* attached to each other, they would be part of the same causal network, rather than merely related by experience or by theme.

To understand the nature of the assumptions underlying the general psychoanalytic theory of discovery of meaning, it is now necessary to make a further distinction *within* the category of "meaning discovered." There are various kinds of causal relationships, different ways in which the psychic entities are attached to each other, and for our present purposes it is essential that we distinguish between two. These two are "*integrated*" causal relationships and "*split-off*" ones. While it may at first seem simpler to discuss these two under the heading of "conscious" versus "unconscious" causal relationships, this would in certain ways be misleading. As we will see, "split-off" relationships and "integrated" relationships may each be either conscious or unconscious.

It is my impression that almost all clinicians have an intuitive feel for what is meant by psychic entities (e.g., feelings, wishes, motives, ideas) that are well integrated in a person as opposed to those that are split off. However, defining these entities is a rather difficult task. To take matters a bit beyond intuition without providing a comprehensive theory regarding them, we may state the following: When the relationship of a certain psychic entity to the individual's other psychic entities is such that each of the two "acknowledges" or "knows" of the other, then we may speak of integration. For example, if my need for admiration is causally tied to my wish to succeed and my wish to succeed is not a blind wish but in a sense "knows" or is "about" my need for admiration—and vice versa, my need for admiration "knows" of my wish to succeed—then the need and wish are integrated. It may also be the case that both my need for admiration and my wish to succeed are causally related to a third psychic entity, such as my love of my mother, in a similar "knowing" or "about" way. That is, both this need and wish may be *about* this love.

It is very important to recognize here that in speaking of a "knowing" or an "about" causal relationship it is not the *individual* who knows. It is not that the *individual* is aware or conscious that the admiration is about love. It is rather the psychic entity, the admiration itself, that "knows." That is, it has the love as part if its content. There are people who have this state of integration who are not conscious of the interrelationships between their mental states, and there are people who are conscious of their mental states but do not have this integration. Integration refers to the state of the ideas and feelings themselves, the quality of the relationship between psychic entities, not the quality of the relationship of the person to these entities.

In contrast to this integrative causal relationship between psychic entities there is the split-off relationship. Here the psychic entities are indeed "blind" to each other. If my wish to succeed is not *about* my need for admiration, if it does not "know" this wish, then it stands outside the interactive integrated causal psychic network. It too will exert a causal influence on the network, but the influence will be different. Integrated entities, because of their interconnectedness, will exert an influence that is in tune with the wishes, desires, feelings, and so on of the person as a whole. In contrast, split-off entities, standing as they do outside the causal interactive network, will drive the individual like a foreign force.

More would be needed to know what *exactly* it means for one mental entity to "know" about another, or for one to be "blind" to another, but for the present purposes this is sufficient. In the course of the coming pages further elucidation will be possible.

I turn now to the discussion of the assumptions underlying the general psychoanalytic theory of discovery of meaning. In this discussion, and later as well, I will refer to the network of psychic entities that are tied together by integrated connections as the "*integrated network of meaning*," or in brief the "*network of meaning*." The psychic entities belonging to this network will be referred to as "*integrated meanings*" and those entities that maintain split-off ties to it will be referred to as "*split-off meanings*."[1]

Three Basic Assumptions

Assumption 1: The Assumption of Effective and Rational Communication of Intentions

This first assumption refers to the way in which the meanings of the individual's network find expression. It is essential for the psychoanalytic method primarily because of what it tells us regarding the way in which meaning may be discerned. According to this assumption, the individual wishes or tends to act and communicate in a way that most effectively and rationally expresses his or her intentions. We always, even in the case of the severe psychotic, maintain that the individual in his or her expressive activity is trying to communicate something; at least part of the person is trying to efficiently convey his or her wishes, needs, and opinions. Our awareness of distortions, gaps, inappropriate affect, and so on, but also of shifts in themes, digressions, repetitions, choice and emphasis of words, and so on, rests on this assumption. We can discover the preconscious and unconscious motives and ideas that affect and underlie these and other aspects of what is said, only because we have an assumption that the individual is trying to express intentions in a rational and most effective form.[2] This is why, for example, when someone (intentionally) tells us of being hurt and yet laughs, we can ask the question "why," and we will seek the answer in the existence of other latent motives (pre- or unconscious), beyond those intentionally expressed.

The person's intention need not be conscious. It is not suggested that the person necessarily is consciously aware that he is telling a story of hurt, but it could be discerned from his way of telling the story that indeed this is his intention. It is in the light of his intention to present it rationally and efficiently that the laughter emerges as a divergent theme. (Another kind of example may be found in the way in which symptoms seem to us to be strange and we seek the sense that underlies them.)

This assumption also allows for the discernment of underlying meanings even in the absence of sharp violations of rational and effective expression. It is because we assume that the person is trying to remain close to the theme that he or she has "chosen" that shifts of themes, and the idiosyncratic way of expressing a certain theme (e.g., idiosyncratic examples that are brought to illustrate a point), become significant sources of information regarding underlying meanings that are latently influencing the flow of the discourse. While some of the latent influences may refer to psychic entities that are in an integrated causal relationship with others, other such influences refer to entities that are in split-off relationships. The latter is usually the case when we note sharp gaps in the person's associations and experiencing, inexplicable sequences in his or her thinking, speaking, and feeling, contradictions between ideation and the accompanying affective experience as well as the absence of appropriate affect. These more powerful interferences with the rational and effective flow of ideas result from the drivenness and blindness of the meanings whose relationships remain "split off" from the broad interactive network.

This assumption must always be maintained in all applications of the psychoanalytic method because it is the search for the intention that guides the discernment of meaning. That is, meaning is seen in terms and in light of the individual's intentions, however concealed these may be. It is very important to note, however, that this assumption does not imply that all psychoanalytic listening automatically results in the discovery of meaning. Rather, it is an assumption that is necessary *in order* for meaning to be discovered. In practice, certain conditions must prevail for the psychoanalytic method to indeed discover meaning. In the absence of these conditions the analyst may assume that meaning is being expressed, but would have to conclude that he or she cannot discern its nature. This leads to a methodological dimension of this first assumption.

A Methodological Dimension of the Assumption. The assumption of effective and rational communication of intentions refers not only to how meanings of the individual's network find expression and to the way in which meaning may be discerned. It also indirectly delineates the conditions that must prevail in order for meaning to be discovered in practice. That is, the assumption itself is assumed to hold always. It in itself, however, does not always make possible the discernment of meaning. Once this assumption is made, certain conditions are required for the discovery of meaning to be *possible*. If the text whose meaning we wish to discover is of an inappropriate kind, the assumption may still hold and the text may still contain meanings, but we would not be able to discern these meanings.

An inappropriate text may be of many kinds. If, for example, an individual was coerced to say what she is saying, or if there are strong constraints on how she is to say what she wishes to say, then if we relate only to the text without taking into account the broader context that includes these various forms of limitation, then the meanings we discern will be false. Indeed the assumption may be maintained that the expression is aimed at efficient and rational communication of intentions, but in these cases the intention lies beyond the available text. The text is an expression of a broader intention (e.g., an intention to please a bully who is coercing the individual to say strange things to us at random).

More common is the situation in which the text is especially brief (e.g., a single word, or an isolated symptom), so that there is insufficient space in which to determine the direct intentions and the interplay of interfering ones, if these are involved. Here too our first assumption holds, but the conditions do not allow for the discovery of the meaning. What is necessary is a text that is sufficiently broad and open—in the sense that it is apparent that the text constitutes one way among possible others of expressing a certain intention. Such a text may be referred to as one that is sufficiently associatively elaborated. Here the individual's specific elaboration of the intention to be communicated, the unique way in which she tells her "story," are regarded as associations to the intention.

When the text is inappropriate, the analyst may wish to modify it so that it will become appropriate. This would primarily involve its expansion so that the broader essential context may come into play. This would be based on eliciting additional associations to the text. Depending on style and circumstance, this may take the form of a direct request, an indirect suggestion to continue with the flow of the communication, or simply silence, the idea being that the silence itself is an association or that it creates a context in which what will ultimately be said will be a relevant association.[3] In any case, it is only when the text is broadened in such a way that the intentions may be discerned that this assumption in practice allows for the discovery of meaning.

A Further Methodological Consideration in Preparation for Assumption 2. In order to fully understand the next assumption underlying the psychoanalytic method and its necessity it is important to distinguish at this point between associations to the text that contain a clear intentional thread and those that do not. The former kind refers to the situation in which the individual elaborates the text by clearly continuing to convey an intentional communication. For example, the individual may express something through a tic. If all we see is the nervous tic, it is unlikely that we will be able to discern its meaning. The individual may elaborate this obscure text (i.e., the tic) by talking clearly and intentionally about some other text and "allowing" the tic to emerge in the context of this directed communication. If the individual starts speaking about how wonderful his wife is and every time he mentions some latent controlling aspect of hers the tic emerges, we may form some inkling regarding the meaning of the tic from this broader context, relying on the intention that we see that he is trying to convey.

The latter, non-intentional form of association, in contrast, refers to the situation in which the individual elaborates the text by providing free associations devoid of any specific direction or aim. For example, the same individual may start associating specifically to the tic: to the sensation it creates in his face, to a childhood event that it brings to mind, to his first recollection of its appearance, to some current event whose connection to the tic is not at all immediately apparent, and so on. Here we do not have a clear intention to rely on, and yet we may nevertheless determine the meaning of the tic, largely on the basis of the assumption of an intention latently determining the flow of associations. In the shift from association to association, as well as from the tic itself to the associations (e.g., from the wincing of the eyes apparent in the tic, to a childhood fear of being hit in the face), an intentional line may be discerned through which it may be possible to determine the meaning of the tic.

It may be argued at this point, however, that in the case of the unintentional form of association, we cannot know whether the associations that are elicited are indeed relevant to the determination of meaning. In other words—since the tic may be regarded as a split-off meaning—the argument here is that we cannot know whether they are relevant to the connecting of a split-off meaning to the integrated network of meaning. When the associations are directed by a specific intentional line, then the connection between the split-off influence and the intentional line of meaning comes naturally into play. The laughter infiltrates the sad story, and on the basis of our first assumption we assume that an additional intention is activated by the sad story and hence that there is a meaning-connection between the two. The tic infiltrates the story of adoration, and consequently the meaning of the tic to, and in, this story naturally unfolds. Here the tie between the associating individual and the split-off meaning is inherent. In contrast, when the associations are not directed by such an intentional line, when what appears to be split off does not naturally infiltrate such a line, there is the possibility that there is a detachment between the associating individual (e.g., raising free associations to the tic) and the split-off entity to which he or she is associating. It may be that the associating individual is viewing the split-off entity from a distance, expressing what that entity is arousing in him, what his response is to that entity, but that these do not point to a real tie between that entity and the associating individual (i.e., they point only to "meaning described"). As a result one may—by seeking out some intentional line—indeed discern connections between the associations as well as between the associations and the entity itself, but it may be that these connections would not reflect actual connections between the split-off entity and the associating individual, but rather would reflect created ones. It may be that we would know what the tic means *to* the individual in the same way that we would know what his neighbor's tic means to him, or what a Rorschach card means to him, but we would not know its actual meaning. That is, we would not know the place of the tic in his causal network of meaning. We would not know the nature of the actual connections between the tic and other psychic entities in the sense of "meaning discovered." This problem is overcome by the second assumption that underlies the psychoanalytic method.

Assumption 2: The Assumption of Original Correctedness

According to this assumption, split-off entities at one point belonged to the integrated network of causal relationships. That is, psychic entities that are split off were at one point in time indeed "*about*" other entities, were not originally blind forces, but rather "knew" the other ideas and feelings and were "known" by these. They were at one point *connected* to the same network of meaning. Their being split off is a result of a process of dissociation or repression, an attempt to defend against the distressing feelings that the connectedness arouses.

To return to our earlier example, the need for admiration may have been originally *about* the love of one's mother, not only causally tied to it. However, because of another idea (e.g., fear of one's father), the "aboutness" was discarded. As a result, the need for admiration is no longer available to the broader causal network as before; it will no longer interact in a complex way with the range of other psychic entities. It will, nonetheless, exert a causal influence on that network and in a fixed way since being separate from the network it is not exposed to influences. Because meaning is defined in terms of relationships between psychic entities, one may consider the shift from an integrated causal relationship (in which the psychic entity is interactively tied to a range of other entities) to a split-off one (in which this complex interactiveness is absent) as a process of loss of meaning. This loss of meaning is one way of reducing distress.

This assumption of connectedness is necessary for the process of free and unintentional association to be significant. That is, the elaboration of the causal relational context of split-off entities through association is important in psychoanalysis because it assumes that these associations touch and revive the actual connections between the split-off entity and the network of meaning. The associating individual, in putting forth associations to some entity that is split off from him, is not *creating* connections between his network of meaning and this entity, but is indeed elaborating real ties that had at one time existed. Were such ties never to have existed, then there would be no basis for the claim that associating to the split-off psychic entities could revive actual ties. This becomes apparent from the examination of hypothetical situations in which this assumption does not hold.

For example, were a person to feel a sudden surge of aggressive feelings as a result of some form of brain damage (of which she is unaware), free association to this text would never lead to a broadening of the context in such a way that would touch real connections. Since the aggressive feelings are not part and parcel of the individual's network of meaning, the individual associating to these feelings would be *un*connected to them. Her associations would be tied to her network of meaning (which is producing the associations), while the aggressive feelings themselves, the subject of her associations, would not. Hence these associations would not describe actual links between the network and the aggressive feelings.[4] In contrast, in the situation in which there are aggressive feelings derived from an aggressive motive that had at one point belonged to the network of meaning and then was split off, associations arising from the network of meaning would produce a relevant context of associations. It would be meaningful to try to trace the intentional connections between the associations in order to determine the meanings that are involved in the aggression because the associations here would be based on the acquaintance (albeit a presently "dormant" one) between the network of meaning and the split-off entity, the aggression. It would not be forging new paths, but rather rediscovering paths, retracing steps that had, in the past, been taken.[5]

This assumption of connectedness focuses on the connection of the associating individual to the entity about which he or she is associating. There is, however, another kind of connectedness that is not fully covered by this assumption and requires another.

Assumption 3: The Assumption of Cross-Temporal Accessibility

This is the assumption that there is a relationship of accessibility between our current networks of psychic entities (i.e., our current networks of meaning) and those of the past. This assumption is necessary for the contention that specifically in our analyses of our past we are indeed discovering meaning, not merely creating or describing it.

Regarding past events or statements, "meaning discovered" refers to the connections of the psychic entities underlying them to the network of causal relationships that existed in the individual at the time in which these occurred. These connections are fixed at a specific moment in the past, and do not change with the passage of time. I may with time learn more about the connections that existed then—I may have not been conscious of them all, some of the connections may have been split off—but the meanings themselves are fixed.

To be sure, the past may mean to me *now* something other than it did in the past (i.e., at the time in which the event of the past was present). I may no longer think that what happened or what was said was significant. I may in the course of time come to recognize that an event of the past furthered my development rather than hindered it; that what was said actually expressed love rather than hate as I believed at the time, and so on. But this is beside the point. This kind of *current* understanding of the meaning of the *past* event is the meaning of the event "to the observer," rather than the meaning "within the subject" (see p. 24). The subject, the person while he or she was involved in the event, existed in the past.

In positing that our past networks of meaning are accessible to those of the present, in positing that those networks are available to us today, this assumption speaks of the possibility of discovering the meaning *within the subject*, the meaning as it was in actuality, in the past. In the absence of this assumption, our current associations to past events—coming from our current network of meaning—would be detached from those that would have been relevant at the time of the event. In effect, we would be standing as strangers associating and integrating psychic entities belonging to another person. The assumption of cross-temporal accessibility overcomes this by positing that our current network of meaning is tied to our networks of the past. We do not simply impose our present network of meaning on expressions of the past, but rather through our current associations, coming from our current network of meaning, we are in fact eliciting associations from the network of the past, the network that was relevant at the time in the past in which the expression whose meaning we wish to discover had occurred. Our current associations allow for the revival of the connectedness between the network of the past and its expression. The analysis of a past event, even one that goes back to early childhood experiences, leads to the discovery of the meanings that may not have been integrated at the time of their occurrence.[6]

Conclusions Regarding the Nature of the Assumptions

These three assumptions that underlie the general psychoanalytic theory of discovery of meaning all refer to two divergent states of the psyche and the connectedness between them: first, the rational, effective, intentional flow of thought, associated with the integrated network of meaning, and second, those split-off psychic entities that find expression through interference with it (Assumption 1). Originally there is a connectedness between those split-off interfering psychic entities and the integrated network of meaning (Assumption 2). And the state of this network of meaning at present is tied to the state of the network at the time at which the split-off entities were split off (Assumption 3).

These assumptions in effect are saying that wishes, feelings, ideas, and so on, that have lost their meaning to us (i.e., have lost their integrative quality of causal relatedness), and thus act within us like blind foreign forces, are connected to what is meaningful and integrated in us, to what is more directly available to us, in ways such that it is possible to discover and revive the absent and lost meanings through the application of certain methods to what is available. Through the application of the psychoanalytic method to what is more rationally and intentionally stated, by listening to what is integrated in the person, we may hear the influence of the blind forces and may elaborate their connections to the integrated network of meaning. Because of the assumption of cross-temporal accessibility we may do so not only for meanings that have lost their connectedness from our current network of meaning, but also for those that have lost this connectedness in the past.

But another conclusion, highly important to the issue of the discovery of meaning, has to do with the implications of the assumptions for the kind of conditions that must prevail in order for meaning to be discerned. That is, while the three assumptions themselves are necessary conditions for the *possibility* of discovering meaning through the psychoanalytic method, additional conditions—the methodological dimension described earlier—must prevail for the psychoanalytic method to *indeed* yield meanings. The three assumptions, taken together with the methodological dimension, delineate two basic paths through which the discovery of meaning may be possible.

In my description of these paths in the coming pages I will use the term "*text*" to refer to a verbal or nonverbal expression (i.e., symptom, statement, fantasy, facial expression). *The "meaning of the text" refers to the meaning that was contained in the expression (i.e., "the meaning of the statement"[chapter 1]) at the time at which it occurred.* Thus if at present I inquire into the meaning of a past text that I now recall, my concern is with the meanings that were being reflected in the text at the time in the past at which it occurred. At a later point I will distinguish between the meaning of the text and the overt script of the text. The latter refers to the manifest characteristics of the text (e.g., the words that were stated rather than the meaning of the words).

The Two Paths for the Discovery of Meaning

Path A—The Intention Path

Path A is based on Assumption 1 and the methodological conditions set forth by that assumption (I will refer to this as condition 1M). In this path the text or expression itself is sufficiently associatively elaborated in order to discern the intentions that underlie it. In this case we would directly listen to the intentions and to the latent influences on these in order to discover meanings. This is represented in Figure 3.1 by the connection between N2—our current analyzing network—and the text.

Figure 3.1. Framework for Discovery of Meaning

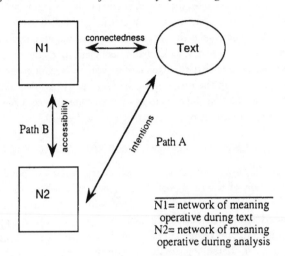

N1= network of meaning operative during text
N2= network of meaning operative during analysis

Path B—The Network Path

This path is based on the methodological conditions 1M and on Assumptions 1 and 2, or on 1M and Assumptions 1, 2, and 3. In this path the text is not sufficient in itself. It does not allow for the discernment of the intentions that the individual is trying to convey in an efficient and rational form. Associations to the text are necessary for its further elaboration. In Figure 3.1 this path is represented by the connection between N2 (our currently analyzing network of meaning) and N1 (the network operative during the past occurrence of the text) and between N1 and the text. N2 associates to the text and in this elaborates it sufficiently in order to discern the intentions that underlie it. In this associative process it is assumed that among the associations are those that N1 would have raised to the text were it currently available. That is, since N1 is accessible to N2, N2 has the capacity to bring up N1's associations to the text.

If these associations take place at the time of the occurrence of the text, then only Assumption 2, which provides for the connectedness of the associations to the text, must be added. In this case Assumption 3, which speaks of the accessibility of the analyzing network to the network operative in the course of the occurrence of the text, is trivial because the two networks are the same. If, however, the associations to the text take place at some time after the occurrence of the text, then Assumption 3 is no longer trivial, but rather is essential to the possibility of discovering meaning.

To illustrate the use of these paths, consider the attempt to understand a fantasy that someone had had some years ago. If the fantasy is very elaborate, we will, in listening to it, try to discern the nature of the intentional theme that is directing it and the nature of the other kinds of meanings (and split-off intentions underlying these) that are influencing the special form the fantasy is taking (Path A). If, however, the fantasy is brief, we will want to expand the context. We may then consider the fantasy in terms of its place within the ongoing communication or we may seek further associations to the fantasy (Path B). In so doing we assume that the associations will truly connect to what underlies the fantasy, although the meaning of the fantasy is unknown to the fantasizer. Also, we will assume that the current associations are relevant even though the fantasy itself is not a current one, but rather one of the past.[7]

CAN THE ASSUMPTIONS BE APPLIED TO THE DREAM?

We come now to the crucial question regarding the possibility of a Holistic justification of the theory of dreams. For the Holistic method of justification of Freud's dream theory to succeed—for the dream theory to be as well founded as the broader psychoanalytic theory in which it appears—it must be legitimate to apply the general principles of psychoanalysis to the dream. This may be considered legitimate on condition that the basic assumptions that underlie the application of these principles in general must be assumed also in the case of the dream. But can they? Can we assume effective and rational communication, original connectedness, and cross-temporal accessibility in the context of the dream?

This is far from obvious. Psychoanalysis's decision to understand the individual in all *wakeful contexts* through the application of these three assumptions is not without reason. We will soon go more deeply into this issue, but for the present the rationale may be roughly stated as follows: The application of the assumptions to wakeful contexts does not stand in opposition to any knowledge we have regarding our state of mind when awake, and intuitively fits well with much that we do know regarding ourselves in that state. Concerning the first assumption, our introspection gives us good reason to believe that while we are awake we are directed by intentions; that at least it is often the case that we do or say things because we intend to, and that our expressions that appear to be unintentional and strange, on further analysis turn out to be determined by certain other intentions. The assumption of an original connectedness fits well with the fact that insofar as we are awake our network of meaning seems to be constantly operative. Since this network is constantly present, the split-off entities may have emerged from that network, and, if so, it is reasonable to assume that they still retain their original link to it. Finally, the generalization of the fact that we recognize and understand ourselves from moment to moment, and generally recognize and understand our past selves, provides the grounds for the assumption of temporal continuity. When it comes to the dream the grounds seem to falter (see Blass, 1994).

The Apparent Special Status of the Dream that Precludes Application of the Assumptions

There are a variety of controversial theses regarding the uniqueness of the dream (Blum, 1976; Greenson, 1978; Kaplan, 1989). In what follows my concern with the special status of the dream refers solely to the way in which the dream stands in relation to the assumptions noted above. I will suggest that the dream has a special status in that it appears that specifically regarding the dream we cannot know whether (1) there is any network of meaning operative, and (2) that even if we assume that there is some network of meaning, it does not seem to be in any way accessible to the network of meaning of wakefulness. This special status is significant because, as I will show, ultimately the evidence that justifies the application of the three assumptions to a given text is precisely this accessibility to the network of meaning of the awake individual. Consequently, the special status of the dream seems to preclude the application of the assumptions that are necessary for the discovery of meaning in psychoanalysis, and thus seems to preclude the justification of the dream theory.

The Evidence that Would Justify the Application of the Assumptions in General

In order to decide whether it is reasonable to apply the general psychoanalytic assumptions regarding meaning to the dream, we must know what would constitute evidence for this, what would indicate that this is indeed a reasonable maneuver. We may begin with Assumption 1, the assumption of rational and efficient communication of intentions. What are the possible grounds for determining whether it can be applied to a given context? Although, as a rule, psychoanalysis considers it applicable to all of our expressions of wakefulness, clearly no one would consider it reasonable to apply the assumption of efficient and rational communication of intentions to an automobile engine, to the regular flow of blood in one's veins, or to statements that are blurted out as part of an organic disorder such as Tourette's disorder. This would be for several reasons; among them the following two are central.

(1) Intentions are expressions of a network of meaning. They are the directedness of the integrated network of meaning. It is only when an integrative network of meaning finds expressions that we have intentional states.[8] If

such a network is not operative and specifically responsible for the expression in question—as in the examples above—we cannot speak of intentions. In all (normal) wakeful states, in contrast, we have good reason to believe that a network of meaning—our regular network of interconnections of psychic entities—is operative. That is why we understand ourselves and what happens around us. We also have good reason to believe that much of our wakeful expression is intentionally determined by that network, inasmuch as we do not usually feel that what we are expressing is strange to us. We may observe the consistency and directedness of our behavior. It should be noted here that these observations strongly rely on a broader understanding of the individual's meaning relationships and on the broader context within which his or her expression appears. For example, if we tell a friend that we would like to cheer her up, and then we say something that appears to be a kind of thing that would normally cheer one up, then in concluding that (at least on some level) there is an intention to cheer, we are relying on a basic understanding of the meaning of what is being said as well as on subsequent contextual information.

(2) Our introspection leads us to directly recognize the intentions that underlie our expressions. Here it should be noted that we must rely on Assumption 3, the assumption of cross-temporal accessibility, in order for this introspection to be relevant. That assumption speaks of the connection between the network of meaning operative at the time of the occurrence of the text and that which is operative at the time of the introspection, analysis, or association to it. For our introspection into the intentions in a certain text or event to have any significance we must assume a connection between the network of meaning operative at the time of the introspection and what was perhaps present during the occurrence of the text.

Thus, both kinds of evidence that would make the application of this first assumption reasonable refer to the presence of a network of meaning. The first kind relates to the very presence of such a network, and the second to a connection between that network and the network observing it. In the latter case, what the observing network would observe are intentions.

We may now turn to the second assumption, the assumption of original connectedness. What is the evidence that warrants its application? Here the relevance of the presence of a network of meaning is even more direct and specific. There is the possibility of an original and inherent connectedness between a network of meaning and a split-off meaning, if there is evidence of the presence of that network at the time at which the split-off meaning appeared. If we know the network was present at the time of the appearance of the split-off meaning, it would mean that it is possible that, although we do not immediately understand this split-off meaning, it nevertheless, originated in that network. If this were the case, the network of meaning would be "observing" the meaning as it was split from it and consequently in some way would be retaining a form of connectedness to it. Thus, we may assume that a symptom has an original tie to the network of meaning since we may recognize the meaningful context from which it may have been split. (In analogy, if we were to misplace something while we were awake, we may assume that we know something about its where-abouts even if we are not conscious of its current location.) Even prior to the recognition of the specific meaningful context from which it was cut off, it is reasonable (for the reasons stated regarding the previous assumption) to posit that our network of meaning was present at the moment in which this occurred. The same is true regarding other of our expressions that seem to be foreign. The evidence of our general and natural[9] coherence to ourselves, together with knowledge regarding the state of our network of meaning that is derived from introspection, gives us good reason to believe that our network of meaning was active even during the occurrence of such foreign expressions and hence the meaning underlying these expressions had been, at least at some point in time, inherently connected to our network of meaning and is consequently accessible to it.

The third assumption, the assumption of cross-temporal accessibility, also has similar grounds for its application. Here what must be shown is that there is reason to believe that the network of meaning that is presently observing, associating to, interpreting, and so on, a certain text has some accessibility to the one that was present at the time of the original occurrence of the text. The evidence for this may be found in the continuity that exists between the individual's present network of meaning and those of his or her past. This continuity is both immediately experiential as well as based on introspection and the observation of the fact that we understand and know ourselves from moment to moment. We do not often look at something we said a minute ago and wonder what it is we could have meant. Our attitudes and beliefs do not undergo abrupt and inexplicable shifts. Also relevant to the proposition that there is accessibility across time is the fact that events that occurred during the presence of our net-work of meaning at a specific moment in time shape the nature of our network of meaning at a later time. Events that occurred in the past, during the presence of the network of meaning that existed at that point in time, have an impact on the network of meaning that evolves in the future. If we are hurt by a figure of authority at a certain moment, this will influence the way in which we will con-strue the meaning of authoritative figures in the future. More generally, interac-tions of the past, thoughts we thought in the past, decisions we made in the past, all these have a real impact on our current network of meaning. Even the fact of having a fantasy influences the subsequent network (e.g., in feelings of guilt, avoidance, or pleasure that are immediately and meaningfully tied to the fantasy itself).

Since our present network of meaning is continuous with that which existed a moment ago, and that network with the one that preceded it the moment before that, and so on, we may conclude that cross-temporal accessibility exists. It may be seen that the evidence that this assumption requires for its application to a given context is evidence that pertains not only to the presence of some network of meaning, but rather to the presence of a network of meaning that is available or accessible to our current analyzing network.

In sum, the evidence that is required to support all three assumptions pertains to the nature of the presence of a network of meaning in the dream and/or in relationship to it. For the first assumption the evidence must point to the presence of a network of meaning *in* the text itself; for the second assumption it must point to the presence of a network of meaning *during* the occurrence of the text whose meaning we wish to understand, and finally, in the third assumption, the evidence must point to the *accessibility* to the analyzing network of meaning of the network of meaning in the text or during it. In wakefulness there is evidence for all these.

To further address the question of the possibility of discovery of meaning it would have to be shown that at least sometimes during wakefulness the methodological conditions that are required for the discovery of meaning—that is, that the text must be broad and open or sufficiently associatively elaborated—are present. Otherwise we would have to conclude that the necessary assumptions for the discovery of meaning exist but that, nevertheless, meaning can never be discovered because we never have a text appropriate for the application of the assumptions. Regarding texts expressed in wakefulness, however, it is easy to show that this is not the case. The very fact that in many of our expressions we can immediately discern some basic intentions points to the fact that the conditions for the applications of both Paths A and/or B to the discovery of meaning are usually available. As we noted earlier, it is possible to discern these intentions both through introspection and observation.

The Question of Evidence for the Application of the Assumptions to the Dream

We turn now to the question of whether there is evidence supporting the application of psychoanalysis's general assumptions regarding the discovery of meaning to the context of the dream. Here matters become considerably more complex. As we will see, when the assumptions are applied to the context of the dream they take on a special and more complicated form. This is because of two facts regarding the dream that we must deal with: (1) the possibility that another network of meaning is operative in the dreamer, one that differs from that operative in the wakeful person; and (2) that there is no possibility of exploring the meaning of the dream during the dream, only after it. This is in contrast to the wakeful state in which there are two potential moments of examination of any given expression—at the time of the expression and following it. Thus, uniquely in the case of the dream it is possible that two networks of meaning are involved, and there is only one potential moment of examining the meaning of what is being expressed. In the following pages we will expand on the nature of this unique situation and how it affects the application to the dream of each of psychoanalysis's general assumptions that underlie the discovery of meaning. We will then turn to see the implications of these effects on the issue of evidence for the applicability of these assumptions to the dream.

The Application to the Dream of Psychoanalysis's General Assumptions Regarding the Discovery of Meaning

The application to the dream of the first assumption underlying psychoanalysis's general approach to the discovery of meaning would mean that we are to assume that the dream in and of itself is a rational and efficient communication of intentions.

It is important to note, however, that here there is the possibility that the network of meaning of the dream is not the regular network of meaning of the awake individual, but rather is a different network that comes into play only in the course of the dream. In this case the meanings that would possibly be discovered from the interpretation of the dream would not be meanings that are relevant to the wakeful individual.[10]

However, since the discovery of irrelevant meanings is nevertheless the discovery of meaning, this possibility of the dream being a rational and efficient communication of intentions of a foreign network of meaning does not directly preclude the discovery of the meaning of the dream. It does, nevertheless, have problematic implications for the possibilities both of determining whether *any* network of meaning is present during the dream, and also for the possibility of discovering meaning through Path A—that is, through the attunement to the intentions. We shall soon see why.

The second assumption, when applied to the dream, refers to an original connectedness between the network of meaning that analyzes the dream and the dream as a representation of some split-off meaning. Only if we assume that the dream once belonged to the (wakeful) analyzing network would it be possible for the associations to the dream to be relevant and to lead to the integration of the lost meaning. While this may seem to be completely in line with the application of the second assumption to wakeful contexts, it should be recognized that it nevertheless differs from its application to all other contexts in one important way: It must always come together with Assumption 3, the assumption of cross-temporal accessibility. This is because, as noted briefly before, uniquely regarding the dream there are never two potential moments in time in which the text in question may be observed and associated to. We may refer to the two moments available for observation and association to wakeful texts as N1 (the moment at which the text occurs) and N2 (some time after the expression of the text). In relation to the dream, observation and association can take place only some time after the dream, that is, in wakefulness (N2).[11] Since we cannot analyze the dream while we are having it—the network active during the dream (N1) cannot be put to this end—in applying the second assumption, we must assume not only a connection between the dream and some network of meaning that was present at the time of the dream, but also a connection across time—between the network of meaning at the time the dream was dreamt, and at the time of its analysis in wakefulness (Assumption 3). We must assume here that the dream belongs to the network of meaning of the awake individual.

But when we come to consider the application of Assumption 3 to the dream, we see that here too this is more complex than its application to texts that occur in wakefulness. When exploring a dream (i.e., a *dreamt* text), I have no access that is independent of the text of my dream, to my network of meaning at the time of the dream. All I have available to me is the text of the dream, from which I might try to reconstruct the network of meaning that was present during the dream (N1). In contrast, when exploring a past *wakeful* text (e.g., a childhood trauma), I *do* have access to the network of meaning at the time in which the text occurred (N1) that is independent of that text. Through memories, I can (at least to some degree) reconstruct the child I was and the network of meanings I had back then, and only then deal with the text in question (i.e., the trauma). Thus, while I can examine a wakeful past text through the past text through the past network of meaning—   N1 (past) ⟶ Text

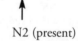

N2 (present)

I can examine last night's dream only on its own, since I have no independent access to the dreamer: N1 (past)   Text

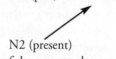

N2 (present)

The network of meaning of the past stands as an intervening entity between our associations to our expressions as a child and the expression itself. In the context of the dream this intervening entity, though possibly there, and even possibly foreign to our current network, is absent to our view or consideration. As a result, when we associate to the dream from the position of our wakeful network of meaning, it is as if there were no dream network. We have only our current associations to the dream that was dreamt, not associations to how the dream would have been perceived from the perspective of the network of meaning of the dream that was present during the dream. For we have no independent access to this network.

The consequence of this special constellation is that the third assumption, the assumption of cross-temporal accessibility, must point not only to the accessibility of the network of meaning during the dream (N1) to the network of meaning that is analyzing the dream in wakefulness (N2). Rather, it must, more specifically point to the *similarity* of the two networks. In order to decipher the meaning of a dream we must have access to the network of meaning from which the dream emerges. But in the case of a dream we have available to us only one network of meaning, that of wakefulness. Thus it is only if the network of meaning during the dream is the same as when awake that we can decipher the dream. It is only if the associations that arise from that awake network are *similar* to those that would have arisen from the network of meaning of the dream (if there is one and if it were available) could we consider the associations to be relevant to the discovery of meaning in the dream. Only then could we consider the associations to the dream that arise from the wakeful network to provide us with the associations to the dream that would have arisen from the network of meaning present during the dream. More simply put in terms of Figure 3.1: Since we cannot observe N1 independently of the dream, N2 must be similar to N1 in order for N2's relationship to the text of the dream to be the same as that of N1 to the text of the dream.[12]

Conclusions Regarding the Nature of the Assumptions When Applied to the Dream

In the application to the dream of the assumptions underlying psychoanalysis's general method of discovery of meaning the situation differs from that of the application of the assumptions to the wakeful state. Two additional factors must be dealt with. The one is the fact that if there is a network present during the dream, it may be different from the network of the awake individual. The other is that there is only one state in which the dream can be analyzed—the state in which the network of meaning of wakefulness is operative. The consequences that emerge from this situation may be described in terms of the two possible paths of discovering meaning.

In *Path A*, the Intention Path, the dream would have to be sufficiently elaborate to discern the intentions that underlie it. Relying on Assumption 1 and condition 1M, we would listen to the intentions of the dream and to the latent influences upon these in order to discover meanings. As in the wakeful situation, the connection would be from N2 to the text of the dream, but we would have to allow for the possibility that the intentions that may appear in the dream are derivatives of a network (N1) that is fundamentally different from that of the wakeful analyzer (N2).

In *Path B*, the Network Path, the dream would *not* be sufficiently elaborate to discern the intentions that underlie it. Based on the methodological conditions 1M and on Assumptions 1, 2, and 3, the intentions would be sought through associative elaboration of the original dream text. Since there is no possibility of associating during the occurrence of the dream, but only at a later point in time (during wakefulness), Assumption 3 will always be necessary here. Also, since we never have the opportunity to directly observe the network of meaning that may be present during the dream, this latter assumption must be further qualified. It must assume not only accessibility, but more specifically similarity, between the network of meaning that may exist in the dream and that of the wakeful analyzer. Since in the dream the assumptions of connectedness and similarity must always go together, they in effect collapse into one assumption of similarity. This has important consequences for the kind of evidence that is necessary to justify the application of the assumptions to the dream.

The Nature of the Evidence that Would Justify the Application of the Assumptions to the Dream

In the light of our understanding of the special form psychoanalysis's general assumptions concerning the discovery of meaning take when applied to the dream, we now may see the kind of evidence that is required for this application to the dream to be warranted. One of two kinds of evidence are necessary.

(1) *Evidence indicating that there are intentions in the dream that may, at least sometimes, be directly discerned by the awake analyzer.* This would allow for Path A, the Intention Path of discovery of meaning, based on Assumption 1 regarding the efficient and rational communication of intentions and on condition 1M, which points to the nature of the text that allows for meaning to be discerned. It should be recalled that in this case there is the possibility that the meanings that would be discerned would be foreign to the network of meaning of the awake individual.

(2) *Evidence indicating that there is similarity of the network of wakefulness with that of the dream.* Assumption 1, regarding the rational and efficient communication of intentions, would here be covered by the demonstration of the existence of a network of meaning during the dream, and thus, if such evidence were available, the conditions necessary for Path B, the Network Path of discovery of meaning in the dream, would be maintained.

We now turn to see how it appears that the necessary evidence for the application of the general psychoanalytic assumptions to the dream is not available. Relying on familiar sources of information regarding the dream, it cannot be shown that there are discernible intentions in the dream, or that the network of meaning of the dream is the same as the network of meaning of wakefulness.

The Apparent Absence of Evidence that Would Justify the Application of the Assumptions to the Dream

The Question of the Existence of Evidence in Support of the Claim that There Is Similarity between Our Wakeful Network of Meaning and a Network that Is Present during the Dream. In our examination of the evidence supporting the application of the assumption of cross-temporal accessibility (Assumption 3) in wakeful life, we saw how both introspective and extrospective data pointed to the continuity over time of the individual's wakeful network of meaning. Indicative of this continuity were, for example, the facts that our experience and understanding of ourselves generally remain constant over time, as do our attitudes, and that events that occur during the presence of our network of meaning at a specific moment in time shape the nature of our network of meaning at a later time. When we turn to the examination of the context of the dream, however, it becomes apparent that the immediately available evidence does not point to the continuity or similarity of the network of the dream and that of wakefulness.

Introspection points to a lack of similarity between whatever network of meaning may be present in the dream and that of wakefulness. It is not uncommon for us not to have any immediate understanding of ourselves in the dream. We often do wonder what we meant by things that we said and did in the dream. Here the words of St. Augustine noted at the opening of this chapter are particularly apt: "And yet there is so much difference betwixt myself and myself, within that moment wherein I pass from waking to sleeping, or return from sleeping to waking. . . . Am I not then myself?" The experience is often that what happens in the dream is not in accordance with what one believes and knows about the world and oneself; that what happens in the dreams contradicts the way we naturally understand things. In the dream I may act with vengeance toward someone I have realized that I love. I may decide to go somewhere and then find myself somewhere else completely unknown to me. My mother may appear with green hair and I may think it particularly becoming, although in wakeful life, not only is her hair not green, but also I hate that color, and so on. What characterizes many dreams is the unusual way in which psychic entities seem to be connected within them (when we apply our current network to their understanding), a way quite disparate from that of wakeful life.

Another introspective and experiential datum relevant here is the very fact of a breach of continuity in consciousness that occurs with the shift to sleep. In wakefulness our thoughts may wander, and yet we can often trace the flow from thought to thought, or at least note the kind of influences that brought about a shift in the flow. In sleep, in contrast, our minds seem to have lost their flow from their ongoing context of wakefulness. The moment of falling asleep seems to be a moment of departure from our regular continuous flow of our ongoing network of meaning. Thus another potential source of support for similarity does not yield corroborative evidence. Experientially and introspectively the dream does not appear to be a product of a network of meaning that is similar to the network of meaning of the awake individual.

Observation points to a lack of similarity between whatever network of meaning may be present in the dream and that of wakefulness. There are various forms of observational evidence nonsupportive of a claim of continuity between the wakeful and dream networks of meaning. One form is an expansion of the introspective data. It is not only from the introspective perspective that we do not immediately understand ourselves in the dream and that our thoughts and actions mystify us. It is also while standing from the outside, *observing* our dreams, that we may note that the attitudes expressed in the dream are not in accord with the basic attitudes and beliefs that we maintain in wakefulness. We may hate vanilla ice cream in wakefulness and yet find ourselves longing for it in the course of the dream. We may know that dogs have four legs and yet in the dream act as though we fully believed it to be a six-legged creature.[13] A basic disjunction between the networks seems apparent.

But regardless of an individual's personal reflections concerning her experiences of her dreams, there are other objective reasons for assuming that the network of meaning during the dream is not that of wakefulness. Central among these is the fact that there is evidence that during the dream the mind in general is in an altered state of accessibility and receptivity to its productions. It is clear, for example, that the capacity for the control of thought in the dream is diminished and that there are certain qualitative and quantitative differences in the way stimuli are perceived and processed (De Monchaux 1978; Foulkes 1985; Kubie 1966; Peterfreund 1971). Such broad changes in the state of the mind raise a question as to whether it is reasonable to assume that the network of meaning remains unaltered and whether it is not more reasonable to assume that this network is in a modified state as well.

Other observational data nonsupportive of similarity between the two networks of meaning may be found in the lack of apparent impact of the events of the dream on the meanings that we have in wakefulness. In wakefulness, continuity was adduced in part from the fact that events that occurred in the past have an impact on the network of meaning that evolves in the future. But a parallel source of evidence does not seem to be available when we come to the dream. The acts in the dream do not usually influence our construction of meaningful connections—unless, of course, we rely on some specific theory about the connection of these acts to wakeful life. If we are insulted in a dream we do not normally awake and return insult. And if we regard the dream more as a thought than an actual event, we similarly find that we do not feel bound to the decisions and conclusions we come to in the dream, as we do in regard to such thoughts in wakefulness. If we come to the conclusion in the dream that we must go off to Timbuktu to find some possibly long-lost relatives, we do not awake and start packing our bags. And finally, if we regard the dream as a fleeting fantasy-like thought during sleep, it is not clear that the dream in any way shapes our awake network of meaning. As noted earlier, in wakefulness even fantasies affect our future networks.[14]

One may object here that there are instances in which it appears that the dream does have an impact on our wakeful network, that such instances emerge when we have immediate emotional reactions to our dreams. We awake from the dream, for example, with a clear feeling of anxiety. Is this not an instance of the dream shaping our wakeful network? My response is that such emotional reactions are not evidence of the fact that a *meaning* that is expressed in the dream is influencing the network of meaning of wakefulness. To assume so would be precisely to assume what is at issue here. There are two attractive alternatives to this conclusion. One possibility is that the emotion expressed in wakefulness did not occur in the dream, but only in the awake person. Our awake network is reacting to the memory of the dream even though the dream itself is expressing no meaningful connections, or is expressing some meaningful connection of a very different kind than the one to which the awake individual is reacting. For example, a monster may appear in the dream that the awake individual considers very frightening, but that in the dream meant something pleasant. It is only if we can know that it was the meaning of the monster in the dream that aroused the reaction in the wakeful individual that we could speak of the network of meaning of the dream having an impact on the network of meaning of the awake individual. But it is precisely information regarding the meaning of what is expressed in the dream that is missing here.

Another possibility is that the emotion *did* occur in the dream and continued upon awakening. In contrast to the previous possibility this emotion is not created in wakefulness. However, the fact that the emotion passed on from the dream state to the wakeful state does not necessarily imply that the *meaning* of the emotion did. The emotion when expressed in wakefulness need not be connected to its meanings when expressed within the dream. For example, it may be that *in the dream* anxiety was felt in an encounter with a monster. When awake we continue to experience the same feeling. It is not necessarily our wakeful interpretation of the meaning of the dream that is arousing the emotional reaction. We have no reason to assume that the anxiety of wakefulness is meaningfully tied to the anxiety of the dream. For all we know it is possible that in the dream the anxiety meant one thing and that in wakefulness another. To take another example, one may awake laughing from a joke told in the dream, although once awake one may not be able to see anything humorous in the "joke." What we have here is the carryover of the emotion without the carryover of the meaning of the emotion—the meaning of the laughter when awake not being tied to its meaning during the dream, or connected to the meaning of the joke in the dream. It may be, therefore, that the emotion that appears in wakefulness is simply the persistence of the emotional expression that appeared in the dream, without any meaning that may have been contained in the dream being of any significance. This would be explained by the fact that the dreamer and the awake individual reside in the same biological system.

As in the instance described here, for us to conclude that it is the *meaning* of the dream that is affecting our current network of meaning, we would have to know something regarding the nature of the meaning that is expressed in the dream. We would have to know not only that the *overt script* of the dream— both the emotions that appear in the dream and the manifest events that occur in it—affects our wakeful network, but that the *meaning* of this script affects this network. If the meaning of the dream is affecting the meanings of the wakeful network, then we may speak of continuity. If, for example, what is being expressed by the "anxiety-over-monster" script of the dream is an anxiety having to do with a fear of castration by a powerful mother figure, and this is arousing in us in wakefulness an anxiety about the same context of meaning, then we may speak of such an effect. In the cases described here, however, we do not know that this kind of influence is taking place. Indeed there may be instances in which what appears in the dream is in line with our general way of thinking and with what we usually know about the world. But the fact that many aspects of the dream are not like this, are not in accord with our regular network of meaning, makes it difficult to determine even in these instances in which the meanings seem similar to those of wakefulness, that what is affecting us in wakefulness is the *meaning* of the dream per se. What may be affecting us are aspects of the overt script that are unconnected to the meanings they represent or contain in the dream. As previously described, we may be reacting to the script and may be having some carryover from it, without actually being influenced by meanings that exist in it.

This last point will be seen to be of special significance when we come to chapter 5. When I there attempt to show that there is indeed a way to know that what is affecting our wakeful network of meaning is meaning contained within the dream, it will be important to bear in mind that there are forms of influence of the dream on wakefulness that do not actually involve continuity of the networks of meaning.

The arguments set forth in the past few pages point to the absence of support for a claim of similarity of the network of meaning of the dream and that of wakefulness. Earlier we saw how the evidence of continuity of the network of meaning over time *in wakefulness* allowed for the acceptance of Assumption 3 and, together with the evidence supporting Assumption 2, cleared Path B to the discovery of meaning. Regarding the dream, Path B for the discovery of meaning could be opened only if similarity between the networks could be claimed. In the absence of evidence supportive of this claim we must conclude that we do not have a basis for discovering meaning via Path B. The dream may have meaning, but we would not be able to discover it.

There does, however, remain the possibility that meaning may be discovered via Path A. We have seen that the requirement that must be met for this path to be supported as a means of discovery of meaning is evidence indicating that the possibility exists of directly determining intentions in what is expressed in the dream. These intentions need not be expressions of the network of meaning of the awake individual—indeed if there is no continuity between the networks of the individual when awake and when dreaming this would not be possible—but rather may be expression of a network of meaning of quite another nature. We may now turn to the examination of this evidence.

The Possibility of Directly Determining Intentions in What Is Expressed in the Dream. We have seen how for the awake individual introspection and observation confirmed that detectable intentions are often present. The individual can report on intentions underlying what he or she is expressing and we can observe that the individual behaves in accordance with what appear to be his or her expressed intentions. Is there similar evidence available regarding the dream? Do these forms of examination point to the existence of some form of discernible intentions—not necessarily those of the awake individual—expressed in the dream? It would seem that here too the evidence is not forthcoming.

Introspection to the network of meaning present during the dream does not enable identification of intentions in what is expressed in the dream. One way to discern intentions would be to try to use introspection to examine the network of meaning active during the dream, just as one would introspect into yesterday's self in order to detect one's intentions. As we saw in our examination of the wakeful state, for introspection into what was intended in a past expression to be of value, we must rely on the accessibility of the introspecting network to the network of meaning present during the expression. In the context of the dream this would mean that there must be similarity between the network of meaning that may be present in the dream and the network of meaning of wakefulness. But we have just seen how such similarity appears to be without basis.

Observation of the script of the dream does not point to the possibility of directly determining intentions in what is expressed in the dream. As we saw in our examination of the wakeful state, in order to determine the presence of intentions and identify them via observation we would have to strongly rely on a broader understanding of the individual's meaning relationships and on the broader context within which his or her expression appears. If we do not have grounds to believe that we have a basic understanding of what is being expressed, and if we do not have access to the broader context of the expression, then we will not be able to identify intentions. If, for example, a person utters the sentence: "I would like to go to Europe," but we do not understand how this utterance relates to the rest of her psychic life and if we are unable to check the context within which the utterance was made, or whether the person does indeed attempt to go to Europe, then we would not be able to know which intention, if any, her statement expresses. For all we know, she may be a brain-damaged person who utters words mechanically, or she may be simply trying out her vocal chords. Regarding wakeful states this comment may seem to be rather trivial, but when we come to the dream we may see its importance. It is because of the fact that in the dream we are missing this information regarding the expression's context and the person's overall meanings that we cannot deter-mine which intention is being expressed, if any at all. In the dream a person may express such a desire to travel, but it is not at all clear that this is an expres-sion of a corresponding meaningful intention. If the person in the dream then does nothing in the direction of furthering such an intention, if it is preceded by events that do not make any sense to us (e.g., she would like to go to Europe to meet her Chinese identical twin with whom she never met), then it becomes apparent that something in the context that would allow us to see the nature of the intention is absent. There may be some intentions in the dream, but we would not be able to discern them.

Since observing the dream script does not provide us with enough data to determine intentions, it follows that it also does not provide enough data to determine the meanings that underlie the dream. Furthermore, if we do not know anything regarding the nature of the intentions that may be expressed in the dream, we would not only be barred from viewing the network of meaning which underlie them, but we would also be barred from viewing their interplay with split-off meanings as well. For example, in the absence of some notion of the specific nature of network of meaning in the dream it would not be clear how one could speak of a gap in associations, an inexplicable sequence of thought or feeling, or a contradiction between ideation and affective experi-ence. Could we define as surprising any transition from one thought to the next, let alone wonder as to what underlying motive could have influenced the transition, without an assumption of a network of meaning of some specific kind that is seeking to maintain a unitary and intentional line of thought in a very specific way?

It is important to reiterate here that the fact that it may not be possible to discern intentions under these conditions does not necessarily suggest that the dream is without intentions. It could very well be that the dream contains intentions that are derived from a network of meaning quite foreign to the one of our wakeful life and that this accounts for the absence of apparent inten-tions.[15] But it would seem that without some information regarding the nature of the network of meaning underlying the intentions, as well as the kinds of meanings it contains, the kinds of directions it expresses as an integrated unit, and so on, it would not be possible to determine anything regarding the nature of intentions expressed by it. Without an understanding of the "language" of that network, so to speak, without the possibility of observing the network functioning in a broader context (as we do regarding the network of meaning of wakefulness), we would not be able to say that any specific intention was finding expression in the dream.

Were we to know that the network of meaning in the dream were the same as that of wakefulness, then we would have such additional information regarding the dream and we would be able to discern intentions. It may be seen, in fact, that Freud's dream interpretations are based on this "knowledge" regarding the network of meaning of the dream. Freud assumes a priori that the network of meaning underlying the dream is basically the same as that of wakefulness. Through his notion of the omnipresent wish, which is assumed to be of the same basic nature as the underlying wishes of the awake individual, he emphasizes the intentional aspect of the dream. He could then—as we saw in the examination of his analysis of the Irma dream—indeed consider certain aspects of the dream to be strange and surprising when these did not correspond to what would be expected from the expression of the wakeful network of meaning. But to make such a priori assumptions regarding the network of meaning and the intentions of the individual is to beg the question. What precisely has to be shown is that the assumption of these is warranted. Thus far our analysis has pointed to the contrary. We have seen that support is not forthcoming for the claim that there is similarity between the networks of meaning of the dreamer and that of the awake individual. In the absence of such similarity we could not treat the dream as if it were a special intentional expression derived from a network of meaning similar to that of the awake individual.

At this point it is important to address the objection that—despite all that has been said here—there does exist introspective evidence of an immediate kind that points to the presence in the dream of intentions similar to those that belong to the our wakeful network of meaning. The feeling, often experienced in dreams that indeed one is oneself—perhaps saying or doing something strange—but, nevertheless, oneself, is adduced as evidence of this kind. Another source of such evidence is in the phenomenon of lucid dreaming, whereby the dreamer has self-awareness even of his very dreaming and has the possibility of intentionally determining the flow of the dream.

This objection highlights the specific nature of my argument. Indeed we may at times experience ourselves to be present in the dream in these ways, but this does not in itself tell us of the actual involvement of the network of meaning of wakefulness or of the presence of actual intentions. In the absence of information that allows us to know something regarding the meaning of events and experiences that appear in the overt script dream, we cannot speak of there being in the dream the same network of meaning or the same intentions as those of wakefulness. My response to the objection is thus similar to my earlier response to the objection that there are instances in which there appears to be similarity between the network of the dream and that of wakefulness. Just as in the dream there may be events with emotional reactions and that arouse emotional reactions, we may in the dream recognize ourselves present and thinking, walking, and flying. We may recognize that in the dream we are present and experiencing specific intentions. But the crucial question remains whether the meaning of these actions in the dream is identical to their meaning for us when awake and whether these experiences of intentions reflect actual intentions. We may even wonder whether the meaning of ourselves in the dream is the same as the meaning of ourselves in wakefulness. Here the evidence points otherwise.

For example, it would not be impossible for us to imagine a thought that during the dream made perfect sense in and of itself (with no additional contextual information), but regarding which when awake we have no idea what we meant by it, even on introspection. The thought may be possible but foreign—for example, "Because I was walking I knew that he really loved me." Or it may be unrealistic or impossible—for example, "Because I was flying," or "Because I was dead," and so on. In such instances, we, when awake, are stymied by questions of what we could have meant by "walking," "loved," "flying," or "dead" in the dream. It then becomes apparent that in the dream our network of meaning and our intentions derived from them seem to be, in certain fundamental ways, in a very different state than that network of the awake individual. Indeed it was I who was walking, but what does "walking" *mean*? What does it mean that in the dream I had the intention to walk, if following this intention I reveal no behavioral correlates of such an intention, such as subsequently going out for a walk? The *overt script* of the dream contains experiences of intentions, but this does not necessarily mean that an intention is operative. The *overt script* of the dream contains experiences that seem at times to belong to our regular network of meaning, but this does not necessarily mean that the networks are in fact the same.

The claim that the intentions and the network of meaning of the awake individual are operative during the dream requires evidence pointing to the fact that the script of the dream is based on meaning connections similar to those present in the wakeful individual. Alternately, were it possible to observe the network of meaning of the dream beyond the context of the dream, then we could learn more about the nature of the actual meaning connections and intentions that underlie it. But as we have seen both from our previous examination of the issue of similarity between the networks of meaning of the dreamer and of the awake individual and from our current examination of the possibility to directly determine intentions in the dream, the necessary evidence does not seem to be available. We must conclude that we cannot learn of the intentions of the dream from the fact that we may at times feel these intentions to be similar to those we experience when awake.

From our discussion in the past few pages we must ultimately conclude that both the introspective and observational evidence does not provide grounds for the claim that there is a possibility of directly determining intentions in what is expressed in the dream. Our examination of the claim of similarity between the networks of meaning of the awake and of the dreaming individual closed Path B to the discovery of meaning. Our current examination closes Path A. It would not be possible to discover meanings by simply being attuned to the text of the dream and to the interplay of intentions and other meanings that are taking place through it.

Before turning to the final conclusions that emerge from the closure of both paths to the discovery of meaning in the dream, let us take a look at one more possible objection to the conclusions. This objection is broad, and questions the very basis of the examinations carried out here.

A Final Objection: Are Not the Conclusions that Are Drawn Here Based on the Examination of Particular Kinds of Dreams?

The examinations of the evidence that were set forth in these pages were not based on systematic empirical study of dreams, and yet involved recourse to specific dreams to support or refute specific claims. The objection may arise that my focus on specific kinds of dreams determined the nature of the conclusions. Had I especially attended to other kinds of dreams, then my conclusion would have been otherwise. For example, there do exist dreams in which everything makes perfect sense in terms of our wakeful network of meaning. For example, before going to sleep I was concerned about how I would do at my forthcoming job interview and, in my dream, there I was, still concerned about how I would do at that interview. Were I to focus on that kind of dream, perhaps I would have recognized greater continuity between the dream and the wakeful states, both in terms of the network of meanings and the intentions that are active in these states.

My response to this objection is as follows: I have not denied the existence of dreams that are perfectly in line with wakeful thought, but rather I have questioned their meaning (e.g., whether the apparent similarity points to an underlying similarity in terms of meaning and intention). This questioning involved the study of the fact that there are dreams whose meaning are apparently obscure. The fact of the existence of such dreams is undisputed. Thus I have not actually limited my focus to a specific class of dreams, but rather I have attended to both the overt characteristics of the dream that resemble wakeful thought and those that are unique to dream. Consequently, it is not a bias in my selection of dreams that influenced the conclusions. Were I to focus only on characteristics of the dream that are common to wakeful thought to the neglect of the unique characteristics and the questions they raise, then I would be guilty of a selection bias and the conclusions drawn would be questionable.

A partial analogy to the situation that arises in the present examination of the dream may be found in the study of the nature of communication of schizophrenics. It is not denied that the communication of many schizophrenics may often reveal many characteristics common to normal communication. But it would be misleading to determine the essence of schizophrenic communication on the basis of these. Rather it would be necessary to attend to the exceptional characteristics that are at times revealed and to understand schizophrenic communication, including its normal aspects, in the light of these. In a similar vein, it would be misleading to determine the nature of the network of meaning in the dream on the basis of those instances in which thought processes in the dream appear to correspond to those of wakeful life. But no such misleading step occurs when the focus is on the dream's unique characteristics. Thus, like the preceding ones, this final objection must also be rejected.

Conclusions Regarding the Availability of Evidence that Would Justify the Application to the Dream of the Assumptions that Underlie Psychoanalysis's General Method of Discovering Meaning

Two kinds of evidence would have supported the application to the dream of the assumptions that underlie the psychoanalytic method in general—evidence of similarity between the network of meaning present during the dream and that of wakefulness, and evidence indicating the possibility of directly determining intentions that are expressed in the dream. Our examination did not reveal the existence of such evidence. Consequently, the conclusion to be drawn is that the application of these assumptions to the dream is thus far without basis, and that the two paths to the discovery of meaning in the dream that rely on these assumptions have not been made available to us. Relying on the familiar sources of information that have been examined here, there is no apparent basis to the claim that the meaning of the dream can be discovered through the application of the psychoanalytic method.

SUMMARY AND CONCLUSION

In this chapter we examined whether it is possible through a Holistic form of justification to justify the psychoanalytic theory that all dreams contain meaning that can be discovered through the application of the general psychoanalytic method. Our approach was Holistic in that it did not try to validate the psychoanalytic theory of dream interpretation as an isolated theory but as part of a larger theory. It sought evidence for the application to the dream of the general psychoanalytic principles and technique by way of which meaning is discovered. If this move were found to be legitimate, then the dream theory may be considered to be as well justified as the entire psychoanalytic theory.

In order to examine the legitimacy of the move, we explored the assumptions underlying the application of the psychoanalytic method and the related conditions under which meaning may be discovered in general, questioning whether these same assumptions could be applied in the context of the dream. While there was evidence supporting the application of these assumptions in wakefulness, when it came to the dream equivalent evidence was not forthcoming. On the basis of an in-depth exploration of the familiar evidence regarding the dream the assumptions underlying the psychoanalytic method could not be shown to apply to the dream and hence the method could not be legitimately applied to the dream as a method of discovery of meaning. The present attempt at a Holistic justification of Freud's dream theory failed. In other words, unless new evidence surfaces, unless new considerations are brought into play, the theory would have to be deemed to be without any apparent basis.

It may be seen that at the heart of the failure to justify the theory is the awake individual's inability to observe the network of meaning underlying the dream. We never see the network of meaning of the dream at the time at which it is operative. It is this unique unobservability that creates the possibility that the network of meaning underlying the dream and its intentions are foreign to that of wakefulness and hinders the possibility of demonstrating its continuity and discerning its intentions. Here lies the apparent special status of the dream in terms of the discovery of meaning. The dream may in fact have no meaning; there may be no network of meaning operative during its expression or the dream may contain meaning that cannot be discovered through the psychoanalytic method. But if there were meaning that could be discovered through the psychoanalytic method, if the network of meaning of the dream were indeed continuous with that of wakefulness, then it is this unobservability that seems to preclude the demonstration of this continuity and presence of underlying meaning.

Ultimately we must conclude that while we know that the dream is a product of the mind, and that in its course it at times *appears* that some kinds of meanings are being expressed, the familiar evidence and considerations are insufficient to show in what way our network of meaning affects, and is affected by, the mental event of the dream. Regarding other experiences and productions of mind, our wishes, fantasies, ideas, feelings, and so on, including those components that would be defined primarily as split off from it (such as a symptom or a dissociated thought), we have found ground to assume that they are usually, in some form or degree, accompanied or tied to our regular wakeful network of meaning that tends to express intentions in an efficient and rational form. As we have seen, on the basis of the familiar psychoanalytic considerations, the dream ultimately emerges as a psychic entity that stands alone and apart from any network of meaning that we can know of, and as an isolated entity we cannot understand it—at least not while we are awake.

One may, as Freud did, make all sorts of assumptions regarding the nature of the network of meaning and the intentions that are operative during the dream, and on the basis of these assumptions believe that one is discovering the meaning of the dream. But on the basis of the evidence and considerations examined thus far, such assumptions and beliefs are without foundation. If these assumptions remain without foundation, we would not be able to know whether the meanings that we may attribute to what is being said in the dream are not an imposition onto it, in the same way as the associations of a stranger to my dream would be an imposition. We would not be able to know whether in seeking ties between the dream and our wakeful network of meaning we are not forging new connections between our network of meaning and an inherently meaningless object, such as a Rorschach card.[16] As explained earlier, a stranger's associations may be interesting, and so may be the observation of how we tend to find meaningful connections even with objects that are inherently completely foreign to us. These processes, however, do not lead to the discovery of meaning, but rather only to its creation.

Is There Any Hope for the Holistic Justification?

Although our examination of the possibilities of Holistic justification of the psychoanalytic theory of dreams has thus far ended in the conclusion that such a justification does not appear to be available, all is not lost. Throughout this examination I have stressed that the evidence and considerations that are being brought forth are familiar ones; that we are looking at the conclusions that must be drawn from what is known and acceptable regarding the possibilities of introspection and observation in the case of dreams, and that we are relying on common assumptions regarding the nature of the dream. It was by relying on these familiar and acceptable sources, considerations, and assumptions that we found that it was not reasonable to apply to the dream the assumptions that psychoanalysis posits regarding the discovery of meaning in general, and as a result the dream theory could not be Holistically justified. I, however, contend that there exists another source of evidence, other kinds of considerations, that extend beyond these familiar and acceptable ones, and that the examination of these does indeed provide the necessary support for justification. There is a neglected experiential factor that when taken into account, provides the missing foundations, the missing link between the dream state and the wakeful one, the link that allows for the application of the general assumptions of psychoanalysis to the dream, and thus ultimately allows for a Holistic justification. This experiential factor is what I will refer to as the "experiential quality of meaningful-ness." Thus, while this chapter has shown that the knowledge presently available to us is insufficient for justification, hope for justification nevertheless emerges from the examination of an additional, crucial phenomenon that has not yet been commonly recognized.

Before turning to the examination of that phenomenon and how it clears the path for the justification of the psychoanalytic theory of dreams, there is one further area that must be explored. This is the area of developments within psy-choanalysis in regard to its theory of dreams. In other words, before "saving" Freud's theory we must first examine whether indeed it still needs to be saved, whether there have not been developments over the years within the psychoana-lytic theory of the meaning of the dream that have made the epistemological questions raised here obsolete. Let us turn now to explore the nature of the devel-opments that have taken place and whether they shed light on the issues at hand.

Developments Regarding the Dream Theory and Its Justification after Freud's The Interpretation of Dreams

I feel sure you are impatient to hear what changes have been made in our fundamental view on the nature and significance of dreams. I have already warned you that precisely on this there is little to report to you.

—Freud, *New Introductory Lectures on Psychoanalysis*

Dreams aren't what they used to be!

—Pontalis, *Frontiers in Psychoanalysis*

The term *experiencing* . . . will have to be understood theoretically if one wishes to avoid mistaking it for a reference to the unutterable.

—Pontalis, *Frontiers in Psychoanalysis*

*A*considerable psychoanalytic literature on dreams has accumulated since the time of Freud's 1900 *The Interpretation of Dreams.* While in the past quarter of a century there may have been a decline in the interest this topic arouses (Flanders, 1993, p. 13), nevertheless, a wide range of clinical and theoretical innovations have been put forth in numerous articles, books, and

debates. As a rule, however, this literature has little relevance for the epistemological question that the present study is dealing with.

    This chapter will be composed of three parts. In the first part I will briefly
describe the nature of the theoretical and clinical innovations that have been put
forth and explain why they are irrelevant to this study. In the second part I will
describe the post-1900 psychoanalytic attempts—all of which were carried out
by Freud—to justify the psychoanalytic theory of dreams. Here we will see that
no significant advance has been made in securing a foundation for the dream
theory and that it is still in dire need of justification. And in the third part I will
take a closer look at one kind of development that has taken place in the understanding of the meaning of the dream—the development of what I refer to as
the Affective-Experiential approach to the meaning of the dream. While this
new approach does not directly affect the epistemological question of this study,
it is important to understand its nature. This is because my solution to the question of the study (to be discussed in the next chapter) also relies on the careful
examination of an experiential dimension—the "experiential quality of meaningfulness." In order to appreciate my solution it must be distinguished from
the experiential aspects discussed by the Affective-Experiential approach.

THE IRRELEVANCE OF CLINICAL AND THEORETICAL DEVELOPMENTS TO THE ISSUE OF THE JUSTIFICATION OF THE ESSENTIAL PSYCHOANALYTIC THEORY OF DREAMS

Careful study of the broad body of psychoanalytic literature on dreams reveals
that ever since Freud first put forth his ideas in this area psychoanalysts have
been seeking elaboration and innovation. What is also revealed, however, is that
the consequent additions and modifications that have been introduced into the
theory and practice of dream interpretation do not have a serious impact on the
issue of the justification of the essence of the psychoanalytic dream theory. They
do not affect the question of whether it is possible to discover the meanings of
dreams through the application of the psychoanalytic technique.

    As we have seen in chapter 1, the development of the hermeneuticist
approach to psychoanalysis *does* indeed have implications for the psychoanalytic dream theory. This is because the hermeneuticists' general concern with
the description or creation of meaning, to the neglect of the discovery of meaning, holds true in the context of dream analysis as well (see also Moore, 1983,
p. 40). For them the aim is not to discover the actual meanings of the dream,
but to creatively ascribe meanings to it through attunement to experience and
thematic connections. As Steele (1979, p. 400) explains: "The meaning of the
dream does not reside in some prior latent dream, but in the manifest dream
and the analysands associations to it." This kind of hermeneutic reinterpreta-
tion of the nature of the process of dream interpretation has become especially

popular. Haesler (1994, p. 15) writes that "There is no 'original' or objectifiable meaning per se of a given dream text as a whole. . . . The meaning of the dream [arises] from the discourse on the dream." All analysts would agree that associations and discourse are necessary for the discovery of the dream's meanings, but here it is suggested that the associations and discourse create, rather than discover, the dream's meanings. Once the aim is no longer to discover actual meanings in the dream then there is, of course, no problem with the issue of justifying the theory that the dream's actual meanings may be discovered. Since we have already presented a critique of this hermeneuticist development in chapter 1, and since without reasonable grounds it obliterates, rather than deals with, the epistemological question in relation to the dream, I will not further address it here.

The other developments that have taken place since 1900, both in Freud and in later analysts, may be divided into three basic categories: developments regarding the application of the clinical method to the dream, developments regarding the nature of the dream process, and developments regarding the aim of the dream. The *first category*, that of developments in the area of clinical method, includes all of Freud's discussions of the technique of dream interpretation that were not directly addressed within *The Interpretation of Dreams* (Freud, 1911, 1916b, 1923, 1925, 1933a). It also includes the numerous technical issues raised by later analysts, such as the importance of the manifest content to the interpretation of the dream (e.g., Bradlow, 1987; Erikson, 1954; Greenberg & Pearlman, 1975. 1978; Pulver, 1987), the importance of attunement to the dream's communicative and experiential dimensions (e.g., Bergmann, 1966, Gammill, 1980, Khan, 1962, 1976, Ornstein, 1987) and the importance of considering the dream as part of the ongoing analytic dialogue (e.g., Kanzer, 1955; Klauber, 1967, 1981). One may also consider the debates on the centrality of dream interpretation to the analytic process to belong to this category (e.g., Blum, 1976; Brenner, 1976; Greenson, 1978; Waldhorn, 1967).

During Freud's lifetime, the *second category* of developments regarding the dream, developments regarding the dream process, included some changes in the understanding of the dream that resulted from the shift from Freud's topographical to his structural model (e.g., the greater emphasis on the conflictual nature of the dream). These additions appeared both in footnotes to *The Interpretation of Dreams* (1900) that Freud inserted in later years (e.g., pp. 476, 556), and in some of Freud's later writings (e.g., Freud, 1940, pp. 169–170). Some post-Freudian writers have further developed this point (e.g., Arlow & Brenner, 1964; Rothstein, 1987). Others have more closely examined the place of this process within the individual's general psychic functioning (e.g., De Monchaux, 1978; Kubie, 1966; Palombo, 1978; Rycroft, 1979). But after Freud the most noted changes in relation to process are those that have emerged from viewing the dream as some form of a container or vehicle. In a nutshell, rather than considering the dream merely as a verbal communication, the dream has come to be seen as a special space for projections (Segal, 1986), for internalized objects (Lewin, 1946, 1953, 1958; Pontalis, 1974a, 1981), for containment of feelings (Bion, 1965, 1970) for living of experiences (Khan, 1983a; Winnicott, 1971), and for expression of the state of one's self (Tolpin, 1983).

The *third category* of developments refers to a wide range of aims that over the years have been ascribed to the dream. While Freud first emphasized the wish-fulfilling aim of the dream, he later suggested (and subsequently also retracted his suggestion)[1] that the dream may have the additional aim of binding tensions related to traumatic experiences. Later analysts have introduced additional kinds of wishful aims (e.g., relational ones—Fairbairn [1944], mature ones—Erikson [1954]) and have focused on other kinds of highly charged material that may seek discharge (e.g., experiences of annihilation—Kohut [1971, 1977], all forms of unpleasurable experience—Garma [1966]). They have also emphasized completely other kinds of aims of dreaming, such as evacuation, (Garma, 1966; Segal, 1986), experiencing (Khan, 1972; Winnicott, 1971), mastery (Ferenczi, 1951) and integration that ultimately leads to a stronger and more adaptive ego (De Monchaux, 1978; Greenberg & Pearlman, 1975; Palombo, 1978; Segal, 1986; Stolorow & Atwood, 1982).

All these developments do not contribute to determining the basic issue of whether it is possible to discover the meanings of dreams through the application of the psychoanalytic technique. Insofar as they add new clinical ideas about what can be done with a dream besides discovering its meaning (e.g., that it may be used to help understand the analytic dyad), they clearly have no impact on the issue of discovery per se. And insofar as they are concerned with the issue of discovery, it may be seen that despite all the clinical modifications and innovations the most essential Freudian idea that the patient's associations are necessary for determining the meaning is left intact. The way to the discovery of the dream's meaning is still by listening to what the awake individual, either directly or indirectly, has to say about the dream. Questions such as how these associations are to be elicited and which associations are of the greatest importance are nuances that emerge from the presence of a basic interest in eliciting associations. Since the essential proposition that the wakeful individual, through his or her associations, has access to the meaning of the dream remains, there also remains the basic problem with this proposition that arose from the study of Freud's work. Grounds for the proposition are lacking.

Furthermore, the developments that have taken place in terms of process and aim do not change the very issue of the discovery of meaning. They too merely suggest that beyond the discovery of meaning the dream may be used for other purposes (e.g., as a context for experiencing or projection), and that there may be additional specific kinds of meanings (e.g., meanings focusing on the state of the self). It may be seen that these additional meanings pertain to the "meaning of stating." They provide new broad answers to the question of why the statement of the dream was made, answers that go beyond Freud's original emphasis of the dream's wishful motive. But the same problematic Freudian proposition that the dream contains a meaningful statement that may be discovered through the psychoanalytic method—the essence of the psychoanalytic dream theory— remains without a basis.

JUSTIFICATION OF THE DREAM THEORY FOLLOWING *THE INTERPRETATION OF DREAMS*

Freud is the only psychoanalyst to devote himself to the task of justifying the psychoanalytic theory of dreams. Other analysts, while offering clinical and theoretical innovations, have not made any substantial contribution in the area of justification. Even for their own new ideas on dreams, often no evidence is provided; at most clinical illustrations are offered—the intelligibility of their interpretations being the supposed indication of their truth, as well as the truth of the innovation that lies at the basis of the interpretations (e.g., Khan, 1976). But the more basic question of justification of the proposition that the dream is meaningful and that its meanings may be discovered by psychoanalysis is, as a rule, not addressed by post-Freudian analysts. In chapter 1 we noted Spence as an exception to this rule. But while he does show concern with the issue of the justification of the dream theory, he has not taken any significant step toward demonstrating that indeed it is justified. Considering the minimal attention and effort devoted to the justification of the dream theory, it is hard to avoid the conclusion that the idea that the dream is meaningful and that its meaning may be discovered through the application of the psychoanalytic technique is simply taken for granted. It is not viewed as something that needs to be demonstrated.

For Freud, in contrast, the demonstration that his dream theory is true was of greatest importance. As we have seen, his magnum opus, *The Interpretation of Dreams*, was his most comprehensive attempt to provide such a demonstration. In his later remarks on dreams and dreaming he relies on the fact that he has already demonstrated the truth of the theory back in 1900. There are, however, several points *after* 1900 at which Freud returns to address the issue of justification. These later references may be divided into two basic kinds: later descriptions of the process whereby he discovered his dream theory, and public lectures on his dream theory.

In the *later descriptions* of the discovery of the dream theory Freud places a somewhat greater emphasis than before on the proposition that it is legitimate to apply to the dream the technique which was formerly used only for the cure of neurosis. But while this proposition is given a more central place, little is done to show that it is *warranted* (Freud, 1901a, 1914, 1923). Freud speaks of there being "numerous analogies that exist between dream-life and a great variety of conditions of psychical illness in waking life" (1901a, p. 635), but does not describe these in detail or show why they justify the application of the same method. In the absence of some argument in this regard we must conclude—as we did in our critical study of Freud's line of thought in *The Interpretation of Dreams*—that Freud's comments on the application to the dream of his method for the treatment of the neuroses is merely descriptive of his discovery process. It cannot be regarded—although perhaps Freud did regard it as such—as a step toward justification.

In these later reviews Freud continues to put a great emphasis on his intelligibility or coherence argument. If the interpretation leads to a coherent intelligible statement, then indeed we know that it is correct and that the true meaning of the dream was discovered. It is in this context that Freud introduces his famous puzzle analogy for dream interpretation. ("If one succeeds in arranging the confused heap of fragments, each of which bears upon it an unintelligible piece of drawing, so that the picture acquires a meaning . . . then one knows that has solved the puzzle and there is no alternative solution" [1923, p. 116]). The limitations of Freud's intelligibility criterion for the justification of his dream theory, and of this puzzle analogy in particular, were discussed at length in chapter 2. In his later writings Freud does not procure any new arguments in their favor, and thus they too cannot be considered real contributions toward the justification of the dream theory.

In the other context in which Freud speaks of the justification of his dream theory, in his *public lectures* (esp. Freud, 1916b, 1933a), Freud seems not only to recognize some of the assumptions that underlie his dream theory, but to be more directly concerned with the issue of actually demonstrating that they are reasonable or well founded. Freud here acknowledges that what underlies the application of his method to the dream is not merely superficial analogies between neurotic manifestations and dreams. He now speaks of his having adopted the initial assumption that "this unintelligible dream must be a fully valid psychical act, with sense and worth, which we can use in analysis like any other communication" (Freud, 1933a, p. 9). Freud here begins with the assumption that the dream is a meaningful psychical phenomenon and therefore considered it legitimate to apply to it his technique for discovering meaning in other latently meaningful psychical phenomena. However, as we have already seen in chapter 3, this assumption cannot be readily made. Here too, Freud ultimately turns to his intelligibility criterion for support. The fact that the interpretation process ultimately produces an intelligible meaning supposedly justifies both the initial assumption of the dream's intelligibility and the assumption that psychoanalysis's general technique can be legitimately applied to it.

But at one point Freud seems to go beyond this limited response to offer a more serious explanation of his assumptions. He does this in his 1916 introductory lecture entitled "Dreams: The premises and technique of interpretation." In this lecture Freud begins by putting forth both his assumption that dreams are psychical phenomena and his criterion for the justification of this assumption—the intelligibility of the outcome (p. 102). But then Freud turns to examine another assumption: The assumption that the awake individual has access to the meanings of his dreams. Here Freud appears to touch on the problem of the apparent lack of connection of the network of meaning of the awake individual and that of the dreamer that we discussed in the previous chapter.

Freud suggests that two factors seem to stand in the way of this assumption of accessibility. The first is the fact that the dreamer, on awakening, does not know what the dream means. If the dream is foreign to her, how could she have access to its meaning? Freud overcomes this difficulty by showing that there is another context in which the individual appears not to know the meanings of what she is expressing, but we know that in fact she does. This is when the individual is under hypnosis. Freud concludes that regarding the dream as well, although the individual appears not to know its meaning, she in fact does. The second factor standing in the way of the assumption that the awake individual has access to the meaning of the dream is the fact that even if we accept that the meaning of the dream is known in some unconscious way, we do not know that awake associations will lead to that meaning. They may perhaps only lead to the understanding of current awake meanings, "to a knowledge of [the person's] . . . complexes. But what have they got to do with dreams?" (Freud, 1916b, p. 109). Freud overcomes this obstacle by arguing that the fact that the dream is derived from the individual's mental life makes it reasonable to assume that ultimately these associations will lead to the meaning of the dream. Thus Freud concludes that the dreamer indeed has access to the meaning of her dreams.

It may be seen here that while Freud raises the important question of the accessibility of the dream to the awake individual, and points to what appear to be obstacles to it, his attempts to overcome these obstacles are rather weak. As we have seen in chapter 3, the fact that we do not understand our dreams does indeed raise a question as to the accessibility to the awake individual of whatever meanings may be expressed during her dream. The fact that in hypnosis the individual claims not to know things that she in fact does is hardly an adequate response to the problem it raises. This clearly does not prove, as Freud contends, that the awake individual knows the meanings of her dreams although she believes that she does. All it proves is that the belief about what one knows does not always correspond to what one actually knows. It remains to be proven that regarding the meanings of the dream this belief is mistaken. Also as we have seen in chapter 3, the fact that one's associations may lead to current meanings rather than meanings that are being expressed in the dream is a difficult possibility to reject. Freud's attempt to reject it by relying on the fact that the dream is part of the individual's mental life is to beg the question. The question is whether all products of our mind are indeed accessible to us—even those that are produced during sleep. Ultimately Freud leads us back to his faulty intelligibility criterion as the sole basis for his justification of his assumptions.

In sum, after the publication of *The Interpretation of Dreams* the only analyst to continue to pursue a justification for the psychoanalytic theory of dreams was Freud. Although he relied primarily on his 1900 "proof" of his theory, he, nevertheless, in several papers and lectures put forward some new lines of thought in the attempt to secure a better foundation for his theory. While he does not directly acknowledge this, it is clear that in these later works Freud had, to some degree, modified his approach to justification. For example, at points he recognized that the idea that the dream is a meaningful psychical phenomenon is an assumption, not a discovery that emerges in the course of the dream analysis. He also seems to have recognized to a greater degree that the crux of the issue lies in the grounding of this assumption and others, such as the assumptions that the technique applied to neurosis is applicable to the dream, that the meaning of the dream is accessible to the awake individual, and that one's associations could lead to those meanings. Here we see Freud almost touching on the special problems in discovering the meaning of the dream that were discussed in chapter 3.

But while Freud's questions indicate that in his later works he recognized the special problems facing the justification of his theory regarding the discovery of the meaning of the dream and the need for a Holistic approach in this regard, the solutions he offered were severely lacking. Not only do they do not overcome the obstacles that stand in the way of justifying the application of the necessary assumptions for the discovery of meaning, but they even suggest that he did not fully recognize the depths of the problems that uniquely face the psychoanalytic dream theory. As he reverts to his intelligibility criterion, the real nature of the obstacle to justification that needs to be overcome seems to slip right by him.

A recognition of the special status of the dream and the problem of its accessibility to the individual's wakeful network of meaning may have led Freud to elaborate his assumptions, but in seeking the ground for them he turns to considerations that neglect the unique status and problematics of the dream.

The Affective-Experiential Approach to the Meaning of the Dream

In this section I will briefly delineate a specific approach to the meaning of the dream in psychoanalysis that has been evolving in the course of the past thirty years. Although it clearly has its own stance on the nature of meaning, this approach has not been formally recognized as an approach per se. I will refer to it as the Affective-Experiential approach to the meaning of the dream. For the sake of convenience I will refer to the traditional psychoanalytic approach to meaning with which I contrast it as the Ideational-Textual approach. The reasons for the choice of these terms will soon become clear.

The relevance of the Affective-Experiential approach to the current study does not lie in its contribution to the epistemological questions that have been raised here. Rather, it is necessary to present this approach and understand its essence so that it will not be confused with the new experiential dimensions that I will discuss in the following chapter in my solution to the problem of the Holistic justification of the dream theory.

The Affective-Experiential approach to the meaning of the dream is part of a broader psychoanalytic position, not specific to the dream, that emphasizes that meaning is, in part, an affective-experiential event. This position does not contradict, and usually appears alongside, the traditional psychoanalytic position, which I refer to here as the Ideational-Textual approach to meaning. According to this latter approach, meaning is an ideational event that underlies a given text. That is, meaning emerges through a process of translation of a given text into the connections between psychic entities that underlie it. The Affective-Experiential approach may be found in the works of Bion (1962, 1963, 1965, 1970) and Winnicott (1958, 1971) as well as in the works of some of their followers (e.g., Green, 1967, 1974, 1977; Grinberg, 1990; Grotstein, 1982, 1983, 1984; Khan, 1974, 1979, 1983b; Meltzer, 1981, 1984; Pontalis, 1973, 1974a, 1974b, 1981). It finds its most direct and concise expression in Donald Meltzer's statement that "The emotion *is* the meaning of the experience" (1981, p. 182). In the course of my exposition I will try to clarify what is meant by this statement and this general position, which indeed is often shrouded in a great deal of obscurity.

In the context of the dream, the Affective-Experiential approach to meaning appears as part of a broader interest in the affective and experiential dimensions of the dream in general. As was briefly noted earlier, among the clinical and theoretical developments that have taken place in relation to the dream there is a growing concern with the dream as a context for experiencing and for containment of one's feelings, and there has been a call for greater clinical awareness to the experiential dimensions of dreaming. Masud Khan (1974, 1979, 1983b) and J.-B. Pontalis (1981) are at the forefront of this general approach to the dream. Careful examination of what has been written in this field reveals, however, that there are analysts who place a special emphasis specifically on the relation between experience and meaning. They consider the experiential dimensions of the dream to be of great of significance not only because experience is important to development, or because it is important that meanings be determined in an experience-near way, that is, while the patient is in touch with his or her feelings. Rather, it becomes apparent that *they consider the experiencing of the dream to be an actualization of its meaning.* Here the Affective-Experiential approach to the meaning of the dream comes to the fore. Its adherents argue that it is important not only to understand the verbal meanings of the dream as a text, but also to attain and actualize the dream's meaning through its experience. Masud Khan explains: "A person in his dreaming experience can actualize aspects of the self that perhaps never becomes overtly available to his introspections" (1976, p. 330). Andre Green in a similar vein states that "if we strive for meaning in verbal terms, we sacrifice our interest in the lived experience of the dream and its significance" (cited in Curtis & Sachs, 1976, p. 351). And in a more extreme form Grotstein (1981, p. 390) says that the "actual meaning of the dream is unknowable" through analysis and comprehension, but we may penetrate this "perfection and mystery" through experiencing: "The divine language seems to intercede on behalf of the person who experiences the dream." It is suggested here that there is some kind of beyond-verbal actualization of meaning that takes place through the experience of the dream. But what does this mean?[2]

It is important to reiterate that this does not merely mean that experiential dimensions should be taken into account when interpreting the dream, or that the interpretation should not be presented to the patient in disregard of his or her capacity of experiencing it. Some analysts have indeed understood the Affective-Experiential approach to the meaning of the dream to refer to just that, and consequently have taken offense at the suggestion that the traditional psychoanalytic approach to the dream is neglectful of such basic experiential factors (see Curtis & Sachs, 1976). While it is apparent that this is not what the Affective-Experientialists mean, what exactly it is that they do mean by this experiential nonverbal actualization of meaning remains blurred by nebulous mystical descriptions and explanations (e.g., "The advent of the dream constitutes an epiphany of Truth which descends or condescends to intervene and therefore present a rent in its perfection of Truth" [Grotstein, 1981 p. 365], or, Khan [1976, p. 329]: "There is a dreaming experience to which the dream text holds no clue . . . [O]ne has to work with the *absence* of a *lived* experience in the person, without seeking for its articulation").

In my attempts to come to an understanding of the Affective-Experiential approach I have found the model of meaning that I put forth in chapters 1 and 3 a very useful framework. In chapter 1 we had spoken of how in psychoanalysis meaning refers to a certain kind of causal tie between two psychic entities within a specific individual (e.g., happiness and a feeling of admiration), and we emphasized that this tie need not be conscious, rather its very existence is what makes for the meaning connection. In chapter 3 we made a further distinction within these causal connections. We distinguished between those psychic entities that were well integrated into the general causal network and those that were split off, reflecting two forms of connections between the individual's psychic entities. The first involves an interactive causal tie, and the latter a tie that stands outside the network of causal interactive ties. It was emphasized that what distinguished the two was not consciousness or knowledge of the connection *by the individual*, but rather knowledge of the connection *by the psychic entity*. That is, the significant difference is not in the individual knowing about the connection between happiness and admiration, but rather in the psychic entities "knowing" of each other, their being "about" each other (see chapter 3).

In the context of this formulation of psychoanalysis the psychotherapeutic process is seen to be geared toward the integration of meaning, the integration of the split-off psychic entities into the interactive causal network of meaning. The interpretative process is not merely one of making the unconscious conscious, but of reviving the lost meaning and reinserting it into the interrelating network of meaning. This is what is expressed in Freud's most famous dictum "Wo Es war; sol Ich werden" ["Where id was, there ego shall be"] (Freud, 1933b, p. 80).

In the light of this model I suggest that the Affective-Experiential and the Ideational Textual approaches do not differ on the issue of the meaning of meaning per se. Both consider meaning in terms of causal connections between psychic entities within the individual. The point at which the approaches do differ is when they come to the issue of how split-off meanings are to be integrated. This is not merely a matter of method; rather *the difference is in what constitutes having the meaning integrated.*

What is implied in the Affective-Experiential approach is that *when the individual fully experiences his or her experiences there is integration.* At the moment in which this occurs the connections between the psychic entities are fully revived. "The experience is the meaning" would thus mean that in the full experience of what the individual is undergoing, living, remembering, or fantasizing there is an integration of the meanings that underlie or are expressed through these events. The individual's meanings are actualized through experiencing. The traditional Ideational-Textual approach, in contrast, turns more directly to the underlying connections between psychic entities. In order to integrate meanings the connections between the ideas underlying the events or texts must be recognized. As in the Affective-Experiential approach, here too the recognition of the connection takes place on a "lived" and emotional level. It is not a matter of making the connections conscious. But the approaches differ in that the Affective-Experiential approach sees meaning—that is, the connections between the ideas in *the fullness of a unitary experience*, while the Ideational Textual approach sees meaning in *the experience of the connections between the underlying ideas.*

This is not an insignificant distinction. Let us look at our earlier example of "happiness meaning admiration." In the Affective-Experiential approach this meaning is attained in the full experience of happiness. In other words, the individual's full experience of happiness contains within it the connectedness to the feeling of admiration. In contrast, in the Ideational Textual approach the meaning is attained in the re-experiencing (whether through transference or otherwise) of the *connection* between the psychic entities of "happiness" and "admiration." It is an *ideational* approach because of this focus on the connection between ideas. The analyst listening from this latter perspective will be attuned to how various ideas and feelings are related to each other. The analyst listening from an Affective-Experiential approach will be attuned to the specific experience that the individual is experiencing at the moment. This is not in order to understand to what other experiences it is tied, as may be the case when the Ideational-Textual analyst is attuned to the experience. It is rather simply to allow the individual to fully experience the experience and in this way integrate its meaning.[3]

It may be noted that this understanding of the Affective-Experiential approach also provides an understanding of the mystical form of speech taken by its proponents. I suggest that this form stems from a certain superficial affinity between the content of this approach and mystical experience. Both this approach and mysticism speak of experiences in which there is a knowing that is not directly anchored in anything that is definable in clear objective terms. Both also speak of situations in which there is a loss of distinct boundaries such that in the individual's unitary experience there is a merging of disparate entities. I refer here in the Affective-Experiential approach to the focus on the fullness of a single experience within which the various connections between the individual's psychic entities come together. However, these affinities with mysticism are indeed superficial. The absence of the transcendent Other in the Affective-Experiential approach annuls any real tie between the two. The mystical and oft-times spiritual tones expressed by writers of this approach are thus not only unnecessary but also misleading. There may be intense experiences of unity, difficult to explain or describe in clear objective terms, but from this the conclusion should not be drawn that these experiences are mystical. They are simply expressing psychological facts.

It may now be recognized that the Affective-Experiential approach to the meaning of the dream does not contribute to the epistemological question of this study. It adds nothing to our knowledge of whether the meanings that we arrive at through the interpretation of dreams are indeed true discovered meanings. Moreover, even were one to consider the full experiencing of meanings a kind of discovery of meaning that can take the place of discovery in the ideational sense, it would still be necessary to contend with the epistemological question of this study in order to justify the claim that meaning is indeed being experientially discovered. If we do not know that when awake we have access to the meanings of the dream, how can we know that in our wakeful *experiencing* of the dream we are accessing them?

In sum, the Affective-Experiential approach to meaning differs from the Ideational-Textual approach in that it conceptualizes the attainment of meaning in terms of a full experience of one's experiences in the course of which the underlying ideational connections within the network of meaning are actualized. The Ideational-Textual approach, in contrast, focuses directly on the experience of the connections themselves. Accordingly, to integrate the meaning of the dream in the Affective-Experiential approach is to experience it fully. As such this approach to the meaning of the dream does not have an impact on the issue of whether it is possible through psychoanalysis to discover the dream's meaning. It was, nevertheless, important to clarify the nature of this approach so that the experiential dimensions of which it speaks would not be confused with the new experiential dimensions that I will set forth in the next chapter. In fact, through the contrast with the Affective-Experiential approach it will be possible to highlight the unique qualities of these new dimensions.

OVERALL CONCLUSION

We have now concluded our exposition of the developments that have taken place and have failed to take place in the psychoanalytic theory of dreams. Despite the basic and perhaps remarkable stability of Freud's dream theory as presented in his 1900 *The Interpretation of Dreams*, several innovations have been added to the psychoanalytic dream theory since that time. With the exception of the hermeneuticist approach to the dream, which completely does away with the possibility of discovering meaning, these innovations, both clinical and theoretical, both by Freud himself and later psychoanalysts, all ultimately rely on the basic meaningfulness of the dream and the accessibility of it meanings. The innovations point to new uses of the dream, additional meanings that can be accessed through the clinical process, new understandings of the motives that lie behind dreams (i.e., "meanings of the statement") and of the processes that underlie them, but all of these assume the foundation and most essential aspect of the dream theory, namely, that the dream contains a meaningful statement and that its meanings may be discovered by the awake individual. Also, with all the developments that have taken place—including the more far-reaching one expressed in what I have coined the Affective-Experiential approach—the basic nature of meaning and the basic nature of attaining it have not been modified in such a way that the Freudian conception of these is no longer relevant. The task of justifying the dream theory remains with us. One may even argue that the variety of approaches that have evolved have made this task even more necessary than before. The very fact that opposing views regarding the specific nature of meaning of the dream can produce intelligible interpretations of it makes very concrete the problem with the criterion of intelligibility, a criterion that is often central to the conclusion that the dream has indeed been correctly interpreted.

Freud considered the issue of justification to be of importance. He felt it necessary to demonstrate that the dream is a context to which meaning may be justifiably attributed. Earlier, in the analysis of Freud's arguments in *The Interpretation of Dreams*, we had followed his extensive and comprehensive Atomistic proof that the application of his method of dream interpretation does lead to the true interpretation of the dream. In his later writings Freud relied on that "proof," but also took a step toward the recognition of the necessity for a more Holistic kind of justification. He seemed to suggest that what needs to be justified is the application of the general technique to the dream; that what needs to be shown is that the assumption that the awake individual's associations are informative regarding the dream is applicable to the dream as it is in other contexts. At certain points Freud came quite close to recognizing the obstacles to such an application; he came close to the problems with assuming the accessibility of the meanings of the dream to the network of meaning of the awake individual. In chapter 3 we had discussed this as the major obstacle to a Holistic justification of Freud's dream theory. Ultimately, however, Freud faltered. His attempts to justify the assumptions were weak and in the course of setting them forth the depths of the obstacle to justification that needs to be overcome were lost. He failed to truly acknowledge the unique status and problematics of the dream, and grounded his claim that the meanings of dreams can be discovered through the application of the psychoanalytic technique solely on the intelligibility of the products that emerged from the processes of interpretation. By relying on the inadequate criterion of intelligibility as the foundation for his entire dream theory, Freud, in the end, did not actually secure a better justification for his dream theory than the one he first put forth in *The Interpretation of Dreams.*

Later psychoanalysts have not been concerned with the issue of justification of the dream theory. With the exception of Spence (1981), who notes some of the problems with justification but does not himself overcome them, the issue has been overlooked. In presenting new ideas, analysts will at times show that their addition leads to intelligible interpretations, and at times will show that it is coherent with the overall psychoanalytic process, but more conclusive evidence remains lacking.

In chapter 3 we clarified the nature of the obstacle that stands in the face of the justification of the essential proposition of the psychoanalytic dream theory—the proposition that the dream has meaning that is accessible through the application of the psychoanalytic method. The understanding of the developments that have taken place in psychoanalysis in the realm of the dream have done nothing to clear the obstacle. The psychoanalytic theory of dreams remains challenged. In the next chapter we will return to the obstacle and attempt to tackle the challenge.

CHAPTER FIVE

The "Experiential Quality of Meaningfulness" and the Overcoming of the Obstacle to the Holistic Justification of the Dream Theory

> And the King said unto them: "I have dreamed a dream and my spirit was troubled to know the dream." Then spoke the Chaldeans in Syriack, "O king live forever, tell thy servants the dream and we will show the interpretation." The king answered and said to the Chaldeans, "The thing is gone from me, if ye will not make known unto me the dream with the interpretation thereof ye shall be cut in pieces and your houses shall be made a dunghill."
>
> — *The Book of Daniel*, 2:3-10

*A*s we now turn to tackle the challenge to the dream theory, let us briefly recapitulate what exactly must be tackled. Tracing Freud's justification of his dream theory (chapter 2), we recognized its limitations. I pointed to the fact that although his justification failed, it was possible that the theory would be found justified according to another form of justification—one that seemed more appropriate to the kind of material that Freud was dealing with and the way he was dealing with it, and one that Freud himself seemed to be implicitly applying. In the place of Freud's Atomistic justification, which proved to be unsuccessful, I suggested that the possibility of a more Holistic form of justification be explored. I pointed out that in order for the theory to be justified in this way it would be necessary to show that it is legitimate to apply to the dream the general psychoanalytic principles and technique by way of which meaning is discovered. The legitimacy of this maneuver was examined (in chapter 3) by outlining three basic assumptions on which psychoanalysis's general theory of meaning-discovery rests—the assumptions of rational and efficient communication of intentions, of original connectedness, and of cross-temporal accessibility—and the conditions under which their application will, in practice, result in the discovery of meaning. I then investigated whether these assumptions and conditions can be maintained in regard to the dream. The upshot of this investigation was that there is an obstacle to maintaining these assumptions in relation to the dream. We concluded that the unobservability of the network of meaning of the dream at the time of the dream seems to preclude the application to it of psychoanalysis's general assumptions. I said: "Although we know that the dream is a product of the mind and that in its course it at times *appears* that some kinds of meanings are being expressed, the familiar evidence and considerations are insufficient to show in what way our network of meaning affects and is affected by the mental event of the dream. Regarding other experiences and productions of mind, our wishes, fantasies, ideas, feelings, and so on, including those components that would be defined primarily as split off from it (such as a symptom or a dissociated thought), we have found ground to assume that they are usually, in some form or degree, accompanied or tied to our regular wakeful network of meaning which tends to express intentions in an efficient and rational form." A Holistic justification of the dream theory could not on the basis of available evidence be attained. What was missing for the application of the assumption and discovery of meaning was either (1) independent evidence regarding the nature of the network of meaning of the dream that would allow for the immediate discernment of intentions (this would allow for the application of the assumptions necessary for Path A, the Intention Path of the discovery of meaning), or (2) evidence that would indicate that the network of meaning of the dream and of the wakeful analyzer were similar (this would allow for the application of the assumptions necessary for Path B, the Network Path, of the discovery of meaning). So far we did not find such evidence in familiar material, but it remains to be seen whether other considerations, thus far unexplored, may supply such evidence.

The challenge we face in this chapter focuses on the second kind of evidence. The challenge is to show that despite the absence of supportive evidence in the familiar material examined thus far, there are grounds for the assumption that the relationship between the dream and our regular network of meaning is such that it allows us to postulate in the context of the dream what psychoanalysis postulates regarding all other contexts to which it applies its method for discovering meaning. If there is a tie between the network of meaning of the dreamer and that of the awake individual, if we can know that the dream as a psychic product is in some way part and parcel of the wakeful individual's network of meaning, then it is possible to apply the assumptions necessary for the application of the psychoanalytic method for the discovery of meaning. It would then be legitimate to apply the psychoanalytic method to the dream in the attempt to discover its meaning. The dream theory would then be Holistically justified. It would be as valid as is the broader framework of psychoanalysis.

As we have just seen (chapter 4), psychoanalysis after *The Interpretation of Dreams*, and especially after Freud, did not make any advances in the area of justification of the dream theory, nor did it change in any significant way that would make the need for justification obsolete. The challenge that faces the psychoanalytic theory of dreams has thus far not been met. I will now show that it is possible to meet it. As I noted at an earlier point, this requires that we take a closer look at an experiential factor that I refer to as the "experiential quality of meaningfulness." I will argue that this experience ultimately provides the missing foundations, the missing link between the dream state and the wakeful one, the link that allows for the application of the general assumptions of psychoanalysis to the dream, and thus ultimately allows for the Holistic justification.[1]

THE NATURE AND PHENOMENOLOGY OF THE "EXPERIENTIAL QUALITY OF MEANINGFULNESS"

The "Experiential Quality of Meaningfulness" as a Quality of Experiencing

In the following section I will delineate the essential nature of the "experiential quality of meaningfulness." This experience is not directly discussed in the psychoanalytic literature and is difficult to describe, much in the same way as the experience of pain is difficult to describe if one focuses on the phenomenology of the experience and does not immediately turn to explain what causes it. It is for these reasons that I will begin by elucidating three basic kinds of situations in which the experience may arise, with only the third one being the paradigmatic situation of the experience. It should be noted here that there are many other kinds of situations in which the "experiential quality of meaningfulness" may arise. I focus on these three because they are particularly useful for bringing to the fore the nature of the experience of meaningfulness. Also, one should bear in mind that the situations described are ones in which the "experiential quality of meaningfulness" *may* arise, but will not necessarily do so—that is, the experiential quality is not inherent in these situations. The examination of these situations will, however, allow us to recognize the unique nature of this quality.

Situation A: An individual has the experience that there is a meaningful connection between psychic entity A and psychic entity B. For example, the individual is thinking about his day at work. The image of his boss crosses his mind and he has the experience that this boss is connected in some meaningful way to his father as a threatening figure. We may present this situation as being of the structure: EXPERIENCE THAT [boss MEANINGFULLY CONNECTED TO father] or more briefly E[b M f].

Situation B: An individual has the experience that psychic entity A has some meaningful connection to something, but does not know to what. For example, relying on the same example from the situation described above, the boss crosses the individual's mind and he then has the experience that this boss means more to him than he is aware of, that he is somehow meaningfully tied to someone or something else. Another example would be that the individual may speak about his day at work and have a feeling that something in what he is saying is meaningfully connected to his father, but not know what exactly it is that is connected. These situations would be logically notated E[b M x] and E[x M f] respectively, where "x" stands for something unspecified (and as before, E = experience, M = meaningfully connected to, b = boss, and f = father).

Situation C: The individual has the experience that something meaningful has happened or been stated, but he knows not what. This is what is described by King Nebuchadnezzer in the biblical book of Daniel from which the epigraph of this chapter is taken. He dreams a dream whose content he does not recall, and yet he experiences that it contained something meaningful and demands that it be interpreted. In this situation the individual is aware of no specific psychic entity that is meaningfully tied to another psychic entity, nor is he aware of even any *single* psychic entity that he experiences as the one that is meaningfully tied to some unknown entity. This situation could be notated E[x M y], where "x" and "y" are the two unknown entities that are meaningfully connected.

These situations describe a person having experiences of meaning connections with decreasing levels of descriptive content. That is, in Situation A the descriptive content of the experience involves two specified psychic entities. In Situation B the descriptive content of the experience involves only one psychic entity; the other is left unspecified. And in Situation C it is difficult to speak of any descriptive content. As expressed by the logical notation, one could say that there is an experience of *something* meaningful taking place, but it would strain matters to speak of this, from a phenomenological perspective, as an experience of any specific content.[2]

It should be noted that what is not mentioned or notated in these situations is the quality of experience. One may experience descriptive contents in various ways—for example, indifferently, quickly, intensely, vaguely, and so on. There may be varying degrees of reflectiveness or immediacy in one's experience. One may also experience *meaningfully*. When the experience is of this kind, what is blatant is a feeling of connectedness of psychic entities or ideas. This is what I call the "experiential quality of meaningfulness." It may be formulated as *a quality of the act of experiencing, the quality being centered on meaningfulness, that is, on the connectedness of psychic entities.* In terms of notation, if the person in Situation A, for example, is experiencing the meaning connection in a meaningful way, we may describe it as follows: E M[b M f], with the first M serving as the adverbial modifier "meaningfully." I will refer to this situation as Situation A′ and when Situations B and C are experienced meaningfully I will refer to these as Situations B′ and C′—their corresponding notation being E M (b M x) and E M (x M y). In these situations, the "experiential quality of meaningfulness" describes a quality of the experiencing of meaningful connections. It is that special sense that something of meaning is at hand, a special sense of there existing some connection between ideas. The person in Situation A is experiencing a meaningful connection and the experience of meaningfulness tells us about the way in which he or she is experiencing that connection.

The "experiential quality of meaningfulness" is not dependent on the descriptive content of what is being experienced. This content may range from completely specific (Situation A), to partially specific (Situation B), and finally to without content (Situation C). In fact, it is in the last situation, when the experience is completely without content, that the "experiential quality of meaningfulness" can find its most pure expression. This is because it is only in the absence of content that the interference of other experiential, as well as non-experiential dimensions, are obliterated. When an experience contains clear-cut contents, then beyond whatever the "experiential quality of meaningfulness," our experiences of the various contents and the connections between them also come into play. In Situation A′, for example, the experiences that the individual has of his father, of his boss, and of the connection between them, will also be present, in addition to an "experiential quality of meaningfulness" that may be present. There also may be a variety of non-experiential thoughts and wishes regarding the nature of the connections between the contents that may blur the "experiential quality of meaningfulness" and even in some way distort it. For example, the individual longing for his absent father may *wish* for there to be a meaning connection between his father and his boss, and the wish may result in pseudo-experiences of connections where there are none. To a significantly lesser extent this is also the case when there is only one clear content. When the feeling is of a certain psychic entity being meaningfully tied to something *unknown*, the interference that comes from the experience of the specific connection disappears, and we are left with a significantly more pure and salient experience of meaningfulness per se (Situation B′). Finally, as already stated, the most pure instance of the experience of meaningfulness emerges when there is no content (Situation C′). Then there is the pure quality of experiencing of the connection—the quality of experiencing meaningfully—without any interference from the experience of the connected entities since in terms of content there are no connected entities to be experienced.

It is when the "*experiential quality* of meaningfulness" is isolated from the *thought* of meaningfulness, the thought of there being a meaningful connection, that we get to see a pure state of the experience not influenced by the knowledge of there being something meaningful. We then also recognize that the experience does not necessarily accompany a conscious awareness of some specified meaningful item. It is not merely a feeling that is added on to the conscious awareness of some definite meaningful thing, but rather may appear independently of such consciousness.

To give another illustration of this more pure instance of the "experiential quality of meaningfulness" we may turn to the analytic situation. There the individual often attempts to follow the flow of his or her associations. But, as we know, these associations flow in a variety of directions and some choice takes place in the line that will be attended to (Kris, 1982). What influences this choice? Introspection at times will reveal the involvement of the "experiential quality of meaningfulness." It expresses itself in the feeling that a certain direction will lead to what is meaningful, that one certain associative path is in some way meaningful. It is not an examination of the content of the present associations that gives rise to this conclusion but rather some sense of meaningfulness. The present content may seem obscure and irrelevant; at times it does not even seem that the present associations are the ones that are meaningful, but rather the meaningful associations are those to which the present obscure ones will later lead. Thus here the descriptive content of the associations plays a minimal part. The individual may not understand the associations and may not *consider* them to be important or meaningful, but the experience, nevertheless, has the quality of meaningfulness. In this instance the contentless Situation C' and the content Situation A' in a sense converge. There are contents present (as in Situation B'), but the contents in themselves do not point to any connection or arouse any feeling of connection (as in Situation C'). There is thus a pure experience of the quality of meaningfulness despite the presence of the contents.

The Judgmental Dimension of This Immediate Quality of Experiencing

In separating the quality of experiencing from the contents of the experience I have been emphasizing that the "experiential quality of meaningfulness" is not a derivative of a conscious thought regarding the existence of a meaningful connection. The thought regarding the existence of a meaningful connection is in fact a kind of judgment—that is, a thought *about* something being the case. It is the judgment or the assessment that two contents are tied to each other. The "experiential quality of meaningfulness," on the other hand, is not *about* anything. It is a quality of an experience, just as green is a quality of a leaf, and is therefore not an *act* of judgment about this or that state of affairs.

Analysis of the "experiential quality of meaningfulness" reveals, however, that one dimension of the experiencing involves an *experience* of judgment. It does not convey an assessment about some state of affairs (i.e., meaningful connections); nevertheless it is an experience *of* such a state of affairs. That is, while the "experiential quality of meaningfulness" does not encompass the assessment that two contents are connected, it does involve the *experience* that they are. As we have seen in the definition presented previously, it is a quality of the experiencing of the connectedness.

It is thus possible to further clarify the phenomenology of the "experiential quality of meaningfulness" by recognizing the relationship of the "experiential quality of meaningfulness" to two kinds of experience, one focusing on the immediacy and contentlessness of the experience and the other on the judgmentalness of the experience. We may take "anxiety" as the prototype of the first kind of experience and the experience of déjà vu as the prototype of the second. Regarding the latter Freud notes the special status of such feelings: "What is no doubt in question is a judgment, and, more precisely, a perceptual judgment; but these cases have nevertheless a character quite of their own" (Freud, 1901b, p. 265). The "experiential quality of meaningfulness" encompasses both the immediate and the judgmental kinds of experience and in this respect is special. But what also distinguishes this experience is the nature of the judgment that it experiences, which is both broad and internal. In the déjà vu experience, for example, the experience is of a judgment that is specific, centering on the proposition that one had been in a certain place before. The "experiential quality of meaningfulness," in contrast, contains the experience of there being some kind of meaningful connection between certain psychic entities.

The delineation of these qualities of the experience will later be seen to have significance for the understanding of the meaning of this experience as well as the meaning of having it.

The Neglect of the "Experiential Quality of Meaningfulness"

I mentioned that the "experience of meaningfulness," as set forth here, has been subject to neglect in the psychoanalytic literature.[3] Although psychoanalysis has devoted much of its efforts to the explication of both experience and meaningfulness, the specific quality of experience denoted by the "experiential quality of meaningfulness" has not been discussed. The explication in the previous chapter of psychoanalysis's concern with the issues of meaning and experience allows for a clear view of where the "experiential quality of meaningfulness" stands in relation to other experiential dimensions related to meaning that have been carefully studied, and how this experience came to be overlooked.

In the course of that earlier explication I had put forth the view that one may distinguish between two psychoanalytic approaches to meaning: the Ideational-Textual approach and the Affective-Experiential approach. The analysis of these approaches ultimately led to the conceptualization of the difference between the two in terms of the ways in which they considered the integration of meaning. It was not that the latter approach addressed experiential aspects of meaning and the former Freudian approach was neglectful of these (as the historical development of psychoanalysis is sometimes misguidedly described [Greenberg & Mitchell, 1983; Guntrip, 1971]). Indeed the Ideational-Textual approach was and is concerned with meanings in terms of the connections between ideas contained within the texts, but what characterizes it in relation to the other approach is that its notion of integration of meaning focuses on a different experiential aspect. The Ideational-Textual approach focuses on the experience of the connections between the ideas,[4] whereas the Affective-Experiential approach focuses on the full experience of the unitary experience. In the individual's full experience of a single experience its meaning are revived and integrated. What is important in the first is the experience of the connection (e.g., that my boss is connected/means my father); in the second the experience of the singular entity (e.g., the full experience of my boss or of my father).

The unique and neglected place of the "experience of quality of meaningfulness" emerges from the comparison of these two kinds of experiences. The experience of the connection in the Ideational-Textual approach is an experience of a descriptive content, that is, *about* a descriptive content (e.g., boss and father). It does not refer to the *quality* of the experiencing, a quality that is not tied to content. It thus does not capture the "experiential quality of meaningfulness." The full experience of the unitary experience in the Affective-Experiential approach also focuses on content, but in addition stresses an immediate qualitative aspect of it—the fullness of the experience. In the addition of this qualitative aspect, the Affective-Experiential approach in a certain way comes close to the "experiential quality of meaningfulness." However, since this approach is not focused on the connection between *ideas* per se, but rather on the unitary experience, the special quality of meaningfulness is not addressed. The "experiential quality of meaningfulness" is a quality of *connectedness* and it is this quality, this judgmental dimension, that is absent in the Affective-Experiential approach.

In sum, the Ideational-Textual approach is concerned with the experience of the connection, but not with the quality of that experience. The Affective-Experiential approach is concerned with the quality of experience, but not with the quality of connection between ideas. The "experiential quality of meaningfulness" is the experiential quality of connectedness, a unique immediate experience of connection, independent of content, that has not been addressed by either of the approaches.

An Explanatory Model of the "Experiential Quality of Meaningfulness"

We may now turn to the meaning of the "experiential quality of meaningfulness." What, if at all, does the "experiential quality of meaningfulness" tell us regarding the psychic state of the individual? What does this experience reflect? From what does it arise?

I propose here the seemingly straightforward view that the "experiential quality of meaningfulness" does indeed reflect the presence of a meaningful connection. That is, when a meaningful connection is in some way activated it may be reflected on an experiential level as the "experience of meaningfulness." If the person is aware of the descriptive contents of the connection, of the psychic entities that are connected in the meaning connection, then this experience of meaningfulness may appear alongside other thoughts and experiences the person may be having about the connection. But the "experiential quality of meaningfulness" is not dependent on the awareness of the connection. It is sufficient that the network of meanings and its labyrinth of interconnections in some way be revived. This may involve the activation of meanings and of links of which we have no consciousness—well-integrated meanings and links, as well as split-off ones. It is the activation of the connection in and of itself that is responsible for the experience, not the reflection on the connection nor any kind of experience *about* the connection.

It should be noted here that when I say that the activation of the meaningful connection *may be* reflected on an experiential level as the "experiential quality of meaningfulness" what I mean by this is that is has the *potential* of giving rise to this experience, though it may not always do so. Whether or not the experience actually emerges may depend on numerous factors, such as degree of attention or the intensity of the connection. In this it is similar to other experiences such as pain, which may at times be aroused by a certain stimulus and at other times fail to be aroused by the very same stimulus.

The Grounds for This Model

The basic grounds for this model are of two kinds. The *first kind of ground* relies on common sense. A commonsense approach would suggest that the "experiential quality of meaningfulness" reflects the presence of meaningfulness, just as the experience of fear reflects the presence of a state that is frightening for the individual, or an experience of hunger reflects the presence of a state of hunger.

The presumption here is that what we experience is usually saying something true of our inner state unless there are reasons to the contrary.

The *second kind of ground* relies on refuting the major objection to this commonsense approach, namely, the objection that the experience may be an illusion. That is, relying on the fact that the "experiential quality of meaningfulness" arises in instances in which we do not see any meaningful connection, in instances in which the individual considers the contents of his mind to be meaningless and yet *experiences* them as meaningful, or in which there is little content apparent to his mind, if at all, one may object that common sense suggests that it is a misleading experience. The fact that the "experiential quality of meaningfulness" arises most clearly precisely when there is no apparent meaningful connection warrants the contention that the experience is not telling us something about what actually lies behind the experience, but rather is telling us that something lies there when in fact there is nothing there—that is, it is an illusion. We are experiencing a sense of connectedness when in fact there is no real connection involved. The refutation of this major objection to the commonsense consideration that leads to the adoption of the model of the "experiential quality of meaningfulness" proposed here, provides further support of the commonsense conclusion. If it may be shown that the "experiential quality of meaningfulness" is not an illusion of the activation of a connection between psychic entities, then the argument that it is actually such an activation is strengthened. To provide the second ground of the model I turn now to counter this objection.

Two Arguments against the Claim that the "Experiential Quality of Meaningfulness" Is Illusory

The Argument from the Absence of an Explanation of the Illusion. This argument is, in a sense, a negative argument. It runs as follows: If the "experiential quality of meaningfulness" does not inform us of meaningfulness and is thus an illusory feeling, there must be some explanation for the appearance of this illusion. In the absence of some explanation as to why such an illusion would be formed we may remain with our commonsense model that it indeed reflects meaningfulness. What, then, could explain an illusion of "experiential quality of meaningfulness"?

One possible form of explanation, the one most significant in terms of psychoanalytic theorizing, is the *motivational explanation.* If there is an illusion of a certain situation, there must be some wish or desire for the situation to be so. Is there then a wish to "experience meaningfulness"? This would not seem likely. If we accept that the "experiential quality of meaningfulness" suggests a connection between ideas, what reason would the person have to experience such a connection if the content of the connection is unknown? The individual may have a motive to find a connection between his boss and his father, but what motive would there be for connecting his boss and something unknown, or connecting between two unknowns? It is this situation of unknown connection that has been presented here as the paradigmatic case of the "experience of meaningfulness."

One may possibly suggest that the "experiential quality of meaningfulness" may be motivated by a desire to please one's analyst who considers this experience to be indicative of progress. This, however, is a weak argument for many reasons. For our purposes it is sufficient to note that the experience of meaningfulness arises outside of analysis and to people who never heard of it. Another possibility is that there is a basic motive to feel meaningfully. Such a motive, however, in the format implied here is difficult to reconcile with psychoanalytic theory because in order to explain the fact that the motive is finding (experiential) expression in a contentless form, one would have to consider this motive to be in some way an *unconscious* one. If the motive were not unconscious, its disassociation from the content of the experience would be strange. This would be similar to an experience of a contentless experience of hatred, which from a psychoanalytic standpoint would only make sense if the aggressive motive underlying it were unconscious. Although from certain psychoanalytic perspectives it may be contended that the person seeks to experience his or her experiences meaningfully, what could account for the *unconsciousness* of such a motive? What undesirable side could there possibly be to the "experience of the meaningfulness" per se that would lead to the relegation of its content to the unconscious? It would seem that the only way that this could make sense would be if one were to suggest that there are certain meaningful connections that the individual would rather not know of, and perhaps for that reason would also not want to experience meaningfully. But then the conclusion would be that if a motive to experience meaningfully indeed exists, it operates in a partially unconscious form precisely because it does activate certain meaningful connections. Thus, in this case too, the experiential quality of meaningfulness would be indicative of the activation of meaningful connections.

It may be suggested that, aside from the motivational explanation, other forms of explanation could account for the illusion of the "experience of meaningfulness." For example, the experience may result from some *misguided form of information processing*. Examination of other experiences that have been shown to have an illusory basis points to the fact that illusory feelings are caused by the misinterpretation of certain cues (Schachter & Singer, 1962). For example, the individual may feel sad because of the fact that his or her eyes are tearing, independently of there being anything really sad that aroused this feeling. Could it be that a similar process may take place in relation to the "experiential quality of meaningfulness"? Such a suggestion falls outside the realm of psychoanalytic thinking, which tends to consider illusion in terms of motive, but it is an important suggestion and needs to be addressed here.

We may address this issue from two directions. The first direction is that of the psychoanalytic framework. From within that framework it would be assumed that even were the experience *caused* by misguided information processing, the resultant experience would nevertheless *reflect* an actual internal state true to the experience. When the person misinterprets him or herself as sad because of experimentally induced tearing, psychoanalytic theory would assume that the experience of sadness still does reflect some internal state of sadness that was activated. The person sees the tears, concludes that she is sad, and then the sadness is experienced because the conclusion of sadness allows for the activation of the internal state that arouses the experience of sadness. This formulation is in line with psychoanalytic theory of affects, but also with common sense. It may be that there are a variety of causes of anxiety and that the feeling can be induced in all sorts of unnatural ways, but this would not diminish from the fact that the experience, when experienced, often reflects the internal state of affairs naturally associated with that experience. (This may be further reflected upon by thinking of a drug-induced experience of anxiety). Thus, even were the "experiential quality of meaningfulness" caused by some misleading information, its presence would nevertheless reflect a true internal state of connectedness between psychic entities.

One may object here that even from a psychoanalytic perspective experiences cannot be considered to be fully reflective of related internal states when additional motives for the experience come into play. If, for example, there is a motive to experience satisfaction in order to avoid the experience of guilt for murderous feelings toward an unsatisfying parent, it would be only partly true that the experience of satisfaction that the individual is experiencing reflects an internal state of satisfaction. It is also, and perhaps more primarily, reflective of a state of dissatisfaction. How the relationship between the experience and the internal state is to be defined in such cases depends in part on one's particular psychoanalytic stance. But in the case of "experiential quality of meaningfulness" this objection is not relevant because of our conclusion above regarding the absence of motives for experiencing the "experiential quality of meaningfulness" unless there is indeed such an internal state.

The second direction from which we may address the suggestion that the "experiential quality of meaningfulness" is a derivative of a misguided form of information processing focuses on the special nature of this experience as not only an immediate experience (like anxiety), but also a judgmental experience (like déjà vu). It may be argued that this judgmental nature of the experience creates a special problem that does not allow us to conclude that even were the "experiential quality of meaningfulness" caused by some misleading information, its presence would nevertheless reflect a true internal state of connectedness between psychic entities. The fact that this experience is an experience of a

judgment (the judgment regarding the actual connection between psychic entities) interferes with this conclusion because the statement that is made by the
experience does not reflect only the emotional state of the individual, but rather
a reality—the reality regarding which the judgment is made. In anxiety, for
example, the experience contains the statement that the individual is undergoing anxiety and that there exists the internal state of anxiety that it reflects.
Since the anxiety is thought to be maintained by that internal state, if the individual is experiencing anxiety, then the internal state is present and hence there
is no room for illusion. But when a judgment is involved, for example, in the
experience of déjà vu, there is a statement that the individual is experiencing
déjà vu and that there exists the internal state that it reflects, but on an other
level it also includes the statement that "I have been here before." This latter
statement is either true or false. If it is false and the internal state that maintains
the experience arose nevertheless, one may consider this to be a state of illusion.
Similarly, it may be that the individual is truly experiencing the quality of
meaningfulness and that that experience is truly reflecting an underlying internal state—the experience of a judgment of connectedness between psychic entities—but that the judgment that the experience reflects is mistaken. Due to
some misleading cue, it may be that a false judgment of connectedness is what
underlies the "experiential quality of meaningfulness" and in this case we would
have to consider the experience to be illusory.[5]

In exploring this possibility we must constantly bear in mind the special
nature of the "experiential quality of meaningfulness." Indeed in its relational
judgmental dimension (i.e., the experience of the judgment that there is a connection) it resembles the feeling of déjà vu. But, as pointed out earlier, it differs
in two respects: in the fact that in other respects it resembles nonrelational experiences (e.g., anxiety), and in the broad and internal nature of the relationship.
That is, the experience of déjà vu contains an experience of a specific judgment
regarding one's actually having been in a certain place in the past. The "experiential quality of meaningfulness" in contrast, contains the broader and more
internal judgment that there is some kind of meaningful connection between
certain psychic entities. This special nature of the "experiential quality of meaningfulness" is what distinguishes it from other kinds of judgments and allows us
to counter the claim that the experience may be illusory in terms of the judgmental statement that it contains. Let us see how.

In the case of a judgment about a specific aspect of reality there may be
some external cue that would lead to false conclusions and to an illusory experience based on it. There may, for example, be some minor detail that is taken to
be of greater significance than it is. The lighting of a certain place, or the smell
there, may lead me to mistakenly conclude that I was in the place before, while
actually I was only in a place of similar lighting or smell.[6] Given the special

nature of the "experiential quality of meaningfulness" we may wonder what would constitute a possible source of misinformation. The cognitive psychologist Foulkes (1985) has suggested that people tend to (mistakenly) attribute meaning to any text that contains narrative, even though the text may in fact be meaningless.[7] This may be so, and there may also be other cues that lead—at times wrongly so—to the conclusion that a given text contains meaning. Certain linguistic characteristics may be of this kind (e.g., the normative use of syntactic rules; [Shanon & Eifermann, 1984]).

But the following points should be taken into consideration: First, the fact that the "experiential quality of meaningfulness" can arise even without any consciousness of the content of the text to which it refers, and usually relates to a specific area of that unknown text, limits the role and influence of such cues, at least of the more obvious and external ones. Even when there is no apparent text at all (at least none that can be recalled) the individual may experience an "experiential quality of meaningfulness." (In contrast to the experience of déjà vu, in which the person usually must be in a certain place to feel that he or she has been there before.) And even then (i.e., even in the absence of any apparent text) the feeling may be that somewhere specific and yet unknown within what has been said a meaningful connection was present. That is, the judgment may be strangely limited to a specific area of unknown contents. Thus, if there is some misleading cue, it would have to be particularly subtle and latent to create such a specific illusion in the absence of any apparent information.

The second consideration to be taken into account is that assuming that there are cues, perhaps very subtle ones, that could lead to the misprocessing of the information, the fact that the "experiential quality of meaningfulness" involves a broad and internal judgment (rather than a specific and reality-oriented one) limits the possibility that it is reflecting a completely false judgment. That is, if we consider an illusion to be derived from the misevaluation of the available information so that in the judgment certain details are disproportionately weighted, then given the broad and internal nature of a latent judgment of meaningfulness, it is unlikely that this will occur. Since a judgment of meaningfulness refers to the very existence of an internal connection, the overweighing of a certain aspect of a connection does not lead to a mistaken connection. Because the judgment is whether or not a connection exists, and the existence is internal, not the existence of some fact in the external world, then even if some aspect of a connection is blown out of proportion (e.g., the similarity between the color of my boss's hair and that of my father), the judgment of there being a real connection between the two would still be true (my boss would truly be connected to my father within my network of meaning). When we are dealing with the judgment that lies behind the "experiential quality of meaningfulness" what determines whether it is a true judgment is not the degree to which it corresponds with specific events in the external world, but rather the degree to which it corresponds with the broad event of connectedness existing in the internal world. This is not affected by disproportionate weighting. There is no meaning to the mistaking of a limited connection for a more extensive one when the sole question is whether some connection exists. (Compare this with the judgment involved in the experience of déjà vu in which the overweighing of a connection leads to the mistaken judgment of having been in a place that in actuality one was not.)

The conclusion to be drawn from this first argument against the possibility that the "experiential quality of meaningfulness" does not reflect an actual activation of a meaning connection, but rather only an illusion of such activation, is that indeed it is difficult to find a reasonable explanation of how this could be. The special nature of this experiential quality limits the possibility of there being some motive underlying it, unless indeed a meaningful connection is being activated. In the absence of an alternate motive the question becomes that of whether nonmotivational causal influences could be responsible for misguided information processing that would result in an "experiential quality of meaningfulness." But as noted earlier, even if this were so, from within the psychoanalytic framework such a caused experience would, nevertheless, reflect an actual internal state true to the experience. The "experiential quality of meaningfulness" is not, however, a simple experience. It is rather a relational experience, containing an experience of a judgment regarding the relationship between psychic entities. As such an additional examination of the possibility that a mistaken judgment is responsible for the experience is also required. This is necessary because an experiential quality may be considered illusory not only if it fails to reflect an internal state of the experience, but also if the internal state it reflects is based on a mistake (as in the case of an experience of déjà vu regarding a place that one has never been at before). Taking into account the special broad and internal nature of the judgment reflected by the "experiential quality of meaningfulness," this examination pointed out that it was not clear what kind of cue could serve as a misleading one in this context, but also that even if there were such a cue, here too, the conclusion would be that the "experiential quality of meaningfulness" caused by such a cue would, nevertheless, reflect an actual state of activation of connections within the network of meaning.

We may now turn to the second kind of argument against the claim that the "experiential quality of meaningfulness" is an illusory experience, an experience not reflective of an actual activation of meaningful connections within the individual.

The Argument from Clinical Experience. In contrast to the former argument which stressed the *limitations* of the view that the "experiential quality of meaningfulness" is an illusion, this argument points to *positive evidence* in favor of the view that the "experiential quality of meaningfulness" indeed is derived from the activation of connections within the network of meaning. Basically I contend here that clinical experience[8] reveals the value of the "experiential quality of meaningfulness" as an indicator of the activation of an actual connection within the network of meaning. If one is attuned to this experience in the course of psychodynamic treatment, indeed one finds that the real connections that underlie it gradually surface. Contents that are felt to be connected for reasons unknown to the patient emerge as significantly tied to each other. And when the contents are themselves obscure—only the "experiential quality of meaningfulness" is clear—the psychodynamic process gradually leads to the emergence of specific contents that are felt and understood to be meaningfully connected.

One may wonder how one can know that the significant ties that emerge in the course of the psychoanalytic process are indeed those that were activated when the "experiential quality of meaningfulness" was felt, and that they were what were responsible for its appearance. Two factors strongly suggest this. First, there is the clinical fact that in the psychotherapeutic situation the significant ties emerge spontaneously, simultaneously with the reduction of the general dissociative and repressive defensive maneuvers. It makes good sense that a reduction of this kind would be the one to reveal the underlying significant ties if such existed. Second, the emergence of the significant ties may be seen to be accompanied by a form of experiential assurance. This is the *feeling* (I stress feeling, not a cognitive assessment) that the connections that have emerged are those that were related to the earlier "experience of meaningfulness." Indeed for this feeling to have foolproof evidential value it would have to be shown that this latter feeling provides veridical information. What I am offering here, however, is not foolproof, but rather only supportive evidence. Consider the experience of having a word at the tip of one's tongue that one fails to recall. At the moment of recall there is a clear sensation of that word (and not other equally likely ones) being the missing word. It may be the case that the experience of "That's it!" has no real value. But we tend to believe that it does. This belief is not wholly unfounded. A variety of considerations support it, such as the fact that the word that is recalled makes sense in the broader context of what is being said, although no cognitive effort was directed to making it so, and the fact that there is no available satisfactory alternate explanation for the emergence of this specific feeling. It is evidence of this kind that I am providing here in favor of the proposition that we can know that the significant ties that emerge in the course of the psychoanalytic process are those that are responsible for the "experience of meaningfulness."

Clinical evidence was Freud's favorite. When he set out to show that the mistaken judgment at the basis of the déjà vu experience was derived from unconscious fantasy, his proof was completely based on clinical evidence (Freud, 1901b). The crux of his argument ultimately rested on case illustrations that showed how in specific instances the experience of déjà vu could be traced back to such fantasies. While I follow Freud in arguing that indeed such positive evidence does exist and is important to the overall support of my claims regarding the "experiential quality of meaningfulness," I do not—as he does—

present illustrations. I refrain from doing so primarily because (as I have contended throughout chapter 2) I do not think that the illustration of positive instances of what I have described significantly enhances the sought-for evidential support. For our purposes what is sufficient is the claim that such illustrations are indeed numerous—they in fact pervade the analytic setting—together with the acknowledgment that this claim in and of itself is insufficient as a powerful evidential basis. For the clinical evidence to provide this, systematic empirical research into "experiential quality of meaningfulness" is necessary. Until such evidence is accumulated the argument that the clinical evidence informs us of the non-illusory nature of the "experiential quality of meaningfulness" is inconclusive, but allows us to go beyond mere intuition in suggesting that this is indeed the case.

Ultimately, the clinical evidence as an argument for the non-illusory nature of the "experiential quality of meaningfulness" should be viewed as supplementary to the argument that it is difficult to explain how it would be possible for such an illusion to take place. Taken together these two arguments provide good support—albeit nonconclusive support—for the claim that when the "experiential quality of meaningfulness" is experienced, some form of connection within the individual's network of meaning is actually activated; that the "experiential quality of meaningfulness" reflects real, not illusory, relationships between psychic entities existing within the individual's mind. It is for this reason that the "experiential quality of meaningfulness" is of special significance for the justification of the psychoanalytic theory of the dreams. We will soon see why.

THE "EXPERIENTIAL QUALITY OF MEANINGFULNESS" AND THE JUSTIFICATION OF THE PSYCHOANALYTIC THEORY OF DREAMS

In this section I will argue that the fact that when awake we experience the "experiential quality of meaningfulness" regarding our dreams indicates that there is similarity between the wakeful network of meaning and that of our dreams. The discovery of this similarity is what allows us to apply to the dream the basic assumptions that underlie the application of the psychoanalytic method to the discovery of meaning in other wakeful domains. Thus it is legitimate to apply to the dream the same method applied to these other areas and to consider what is derived from this application to be "meaning discovered." In this way the psychoanalytic theory that dreams have meaning accessible to the awake analyzer is Holistically justified.

The "Experiential Quality of Meaningfulness" in Relation to the Dream

It is a common phenomenon, at least for many people, that they experience "experiential qualities of meaningfulness" in relation to some of their dreams.

That is, many people do not only consider the dream to contain meaning on the basis of a scientific investigation of the issue, common belief, or convincing demonstration, but rather feel this meaning in an immediate way, without any noteworthy basis. There is an intruding and overwhelming sense of truth that is based not on a learned judgment, or, as noted earlier, on illusion. What is particularly striking in the "experiential quality of meaningfulness" in relation to the dream is the degree to which content may be absent. As in the case of the dream of King Nebuchadnezzer in the Book of Daniel, there may be no content whatsoever at the time of the recall of the dream and yet a sense of meaningfulness prevails. More common, however, are feelings of the quality of meaningfulness in relation to certain aspects of the dream that do not make any apparent sense. They may be an isolated expression, such as a sudden thud, or a clear, yet strange expression (e.g., "I was flying through the air") or a clear and plain expression whose strangeness or senselessness comes from the absence of context (e.g., "I said hello to my mother"). In all these instances there may be an experience that the apparently meaningless contents have meaning. While I clearly know what the words "I said hello to my mother" mean in the semantic sense, it remains obscure what I mean by these words in the dream, why I am saying them. And yet I may experience that they have meaning—not necessarily that I know what that meaning is, but that it in some way contains meaning. What we have here are situations in which the dream, or parts of it, is experienced meaningfully. Since the dream as a whole is in a sense out of context—it is not apparently part of the ongoing wakeful flow of thought that precedes and follows it—*any direct experience* of the dream as meaningful is in effect an "experiential quality of meaningfulness" of this kind.

The Location of the "Experiential Quality of Meaningfulness" in Relation to the Dream

A very important dimension of the "experiential quality of meaningfulness" in relation to the dream has to do with the "location" of the experience. Where, so to speak, is the experience taking place? In the dream? In wakefulness? It may be seen that there are two locations that must be taken into account. The "experiential quality of meaningfulness" in relation to the dream is located in the dream in the sense that it is about the meaningfulness of the dream, it is an experience of the dream. But it is also located in wakefulness, in the sense that it is in the awake individual that the experience takes place. In other words, the awake person now experiences the meaningfulness of what was expressed—back then—in the course of the dream. When awake the individual experiences the meaningfulness of what transpired in the dream. For example, on awakening the individual may experience the meaningfulness of the image of his boss that appeared in the dream.

It is important to distinguish this "experiential quality of meaningfulness" in relation to the dream from two other kinds of experiences that on a superficial level may appear to be similar. The first kind emerges when the awake person experiences the meaningfulness not of his past dream, but rather of his present, awake, encounter with the dream. In this case, the experience is not of the meaningfulness *in* his dream, but rather of meaningfulness in the awake person when remembering his dream. The experience is aroused by the *overt script* of the dream text, by its manifest characteristics, not by the *original meanings* that are in it. For example, upon awakening the image of the boss in the dream is not experienced as having been meaningful, but when the individual thinks how in the dream script his boss resembled his father he *now* meaningfully experiences the connection between his boss and his father.

The second kind of experience emerges when the individual does not now experience the meaningfulness *of* the past dream, but rather now remembers an experience of meaningfulness that had *existed in the past*, at the time of the dream, and no longer exists. That is, the individual had experienced meaningfulness in the course of the dream and whether or not he later remembers that experience, that experience is only of meaningfulness that had existed at the time of the dream. For example, the individual has a dream in which he has a meaningful experience of his boss. When he awakes he recalls this experience among the other contents of the dream. The dream itself, however, is not experienced as meaningful.

In contrast to these two kinds of experiences what is experienced in the "experiential quality of meaningfulness" in relation the dream is not an experience of "*now* I feel something to be meaningful," nor is it one of "now I recall that there was something meaningful then," but rather it is an experience of "now I feel the meaningfulness *then*, that is, of the dream."

This "double location"—the present experience of the past—of the "experiential quality of meaningfulness" is unique and does not arise in the case of other immediate experiences (e.g., anxiety) or other experiences of a judgmental kind (e.g., déjà vu). In other experiences the experience is either in the present (possibly regarding the past, e.g., now I feel anxious about what I had dreamt), or in the past (e.g., in the dream I felt anxiety), but the experience is never a present experiencing of the past (e.g., it is never of the form: now I feel anxiety that is the anxiety of the dreaming experience, although it was not present in the dream itself).[9] In other experiences the experience is *about* the dream (e.g., I feel that I had once before been in the place that appeared in the dream).

In terms of the location of the experiences in the context of the dream, immediate and contentless experiences, such as anxiety, and judgmental experiences, such as déjà vu, are similar. These experiences either emerge in the course of the dream or in the awake individual as a reaction to the dream. They are about the dream. The "experiential quality of meaningfulness" stands apart from these experiences, uniquely providing a situation in which there is a wakeful experience of the meaningfulness of the dream at the time at which it was dreamt. This is, as we will soon see, a highly significant fact for the justification of the psychoanalytic dream theory.

What the "Experiential Quality of Meaningfulness" Tells Us Regarding the Possibility of Discovering the Meaning of the Dream

We have examined the nature of the "experiential quality of meaningfulness," proposed a model that may explain it, and pointed to a special form of presence of this experience in relation to our dreams. Now we may turn to see the impact of these for the possibility of discovering the meaning of dreams.

In our discussion of our model for the "experiential quality of meaningfulness" we had concluded that there is good reason to believe that this experience is a reflection of the activation of some kind of meaningful connection; that when we experience this experience—whether regarding known or absent content—we can know that a relationship between psychic entities that are in some way tied to our network of meaning are being activated or touched. Now we may add to this that when awake we may experience *in* the dream (note the stress on "in") an "experiential quality of meaningfulness." Putting these together we may conclude that *the "experiential quality of meaningfulness" in relation to the dream reflects our wakeful knowledge of a meaningful connection having been activated in the dream.* That is, the individual experiencing an "experiential quality of meaningfulness" in relation to the dream knows, while awake, that in the dream a meaningful connection between two psychic entities was activated. This conclusion has crucial implications for the possibility of justifying the psychoanalytic theory of dreams. Its significance becomes apparent from a comparison with some of our earlier attempts to demonstrate the existence of similarity between the network of meaning of the dream and that of the awake individual. Thus let us briefly return now to some of our earlier comments.

In chapter 3 we saw how familiar introspective and extrospective evidence did not support the view that there is similarity between the network of meaning that may be present in the dream and that of the awake individual. The great differences between the attitudes expressed in the dream and those of our wakeful network, the breach in continuity of consciousness with the shift to sleep, and the lack of immediate understanding by the awake individual of what he or she had expressed in the dream, were among the nonsupportive data. Toward the end of that chapter we had examined the objection that there are various situations in which it indeed does appear that the network of meaning of the dream may be affecting the network of meaning of the awake individual, and thus that they may nevertheless be closely tied. An example of this was the situation in which the individual awakes with a sense of anxiety from a dream either in which there was anxiety, or a situation that the awake individual considers to be anxiety arousing. The closer scrutiny of such situations, however, revealed that while there was an apparent influence of the dream on the awake individual, it could not be determined that, in fact, the *meaning* of the dream was what was affecting the network of meaning of the awake individual. We saw how, in various ways, it could be that the *overt script* of the dream was affecting the individual's awake network of meaning without any involvement of the underlying meanings that may be contained in the dream. Anxiety in the dream may not mean what anxiety means in the awake state. The awake feeling of anxiety could have had nothing to do with the meaning of the anxiety of the dream or the meaning of the events related to it. Thus we concluded that such situations did not indicate that the networks of meaning that may be present during the dream and that of the awake individual were basically the same, or were even in some way continuous. For us to attribute similarity to the networks we would have to know that the *meanings* of the one were tied to the *meanings* of the other.

It is in contrast with these failed attempts to support the claim of similarity that we see the great significance of the "experiential quality of meaningfulness" in relation to the dream. *Uniquely regarding the "experiential quality of meaningfulness" experienced in relation to the dream it cannot be claimed that this experience is a reaction to the overt script of the dream independently of the meanings contained in that script.* Since, as we have concluded, the "experiential quality of meaningfulness" in relation to the dream reflects our wakeful experience of a meaningful connection having been actually activated in the dream, since it tells us that the awake individual experiences that in the dream a meaningful connection between two psychic entities had been activated, we must conclude that it is specifically the *meaning* of the dream that is affecting the network of meaning of the awake individual. *The network of meaning of the awake individual is being affected by the network of meaning of the dream,* not by the overt script. The wakeful network of meaning is reflecting the meanings of the network of meaning that was present during the dream. Note that the point is not that we may judge the overt script to have meaning for us when awake, nor is it that we may recognize in the overt script feelings of meaningfulness, for this is not the "experiential quality of meaningfulness" in relation to the dream. In the "experiential quality of meaningfulness" in relation to the dream the overt script does not play a significant role; it is its meaning that does.

The implication of this is that the link between the network of meaning that is present during the dream and the network of meaning of the awake individual has finally been found. The network of the awake individual can touch the meanings of the dreamer. There is a potential common language between the two. This means that not only does the network of meaning of the awake individual have the potential to comprehend and appreciate the meanings of the network of meaning of the dreamer, but that it participates in that network. The awake network senses the meanings of the network that existed in the past, in the dreamer. *This could occur only if the awake network and that of the dreamer are basically the same.* One can immediately experience the meaningfulness only of one's own meanings (just as one can immediately experience only one's own pain, no matter how deeply one may empathize with the pain of another). *The inevitable conclusion is that the two networks are the same.*

It is important to stress here that the similarity of networks of the awake individual and that of the dreamer does not in any way suggest that one can immediately comprehend one's dreams when one observes them upon awakening. We know that this is not the case. What this similarity does mean is that in the mind of the awake individual and the mind of the dreamer there are the same basic meaning connections. If in the mind of the awake individual there is a meaningful causal tie between one's father and the idea of threat, then this same causal tie exists in the mind of the dreamer. And vice versa: the meaningful causal ties in the mind of the dreamer also exist in the mind of the awake individual. What we have shown here is that the two networks are the same in terms of the nature of their meanings, their underlying interconnections between psychic entities. On the manifest level, these meanings may find different forms of expression in wakefulness and during the dream. The strangeness and immediate incomprehensibility of the dream suggest that this is indeed the case.

The Psychoanalytic Theory of the Dream Finds Justification

Our earlier examination of the dream had shown that psychoanalytic theory of the dream could not be considered to be justified because of the absence of one of two kinds of evidence—evidence of the existence of intentions in the dream that could be discerned by the awake individual or evidence of similarity between the networks of meaning of the awake individual and that of the dream. We have now seen that the wakeful presence of the "experiential quality of meaningfulness" in relation to the dream provides evidence of the latter. Given the presence of evidence of the similarity between the networks, we may conclude that the psychoanalytic theory of the dream has found the necessary basis for its justification. *Quod erat demonstrandum.*

WE MAY DISCOVER MEANING THROUGH THE APPLICATION OF THE PSYCHOANALYTIC METHOD TO THE DREAM

Let us now take a broader look at what we have found through our examination of the "experiential quality of meaningfulness" and explore the implications of our findings. In chapter 3 we had set out to determine whether a Holistic approach to justification may allow for the justification of the psychoanalytic theory of dreams where Freud's Atomistic approach failed. We saw that to use a Holistic approach here would mean to demonstrate that the general psychoanalytic method of discovery of meaning may be legitimately applied to the specific case of the dream; that there is good reason to believe that when that method is applied to the dream, then the product of the interpretative process is indeed discovered meaning and not simply meanings assigned to the dream by the awake individual. We further saw that one way of showing the legitimacy of applying the psychoanalytic method to the dream was by showing that it is reasonable to assume in relation to the dream the same general assumptions that underlie psychoanalysis's method of discovery of meaning in wakeful contexts. If the assumptions that allow for the discovery of meaning through the application of the psychoanalytic method to the individual's wakeful expressions can also be maintained when the expression we wish to understand is the dream, then it is legitimate to conclude that the application of that method to the dream will also result in the discovery of meaning. Having then outlined the assumptions that allow for the discovery of meaning in general we examined whether it would be possible to successfully apply them to the dream.

What emerged was that the application of these assumptions to the dream was not a simple matter. One of two kinds of necessary evidence had to be procured. One kind of evidence was of there being intentions in the dream that could be discerned by the awake individual. If this kind of evidence were available, it could be concluded that while we do not know the relationship between the networks of meaning of the awake individual to that of the dreamer, we could bypass the dreamer's network and discover the meanings that are expressed by the network of meaning of the dream. The other kind of evidence that was necessary was evidence of similarity between the networks of meaning of the dream and that of the awake individual. If such similarity existed then the awake individual's associations to the dream could be considered elaborations of the meanings expressed in the dream and through such elaboration the intentions would emerge and with them the underlying meanings.

In chapter 3 we found the necessary kinds of evidence to be absent, and in chapter 4 it became apparent, through a review of the relevant literature, that with all the developments that have taken place over the years in relation to the psychoanalysis of dreams, the need for such evidence has not diminished, nor has such evidence surfaced.

Our examination of the "experiential quality of meaningfulness" has, however, shown that the necessary evidence is nevertheless available. Through a thorough rational analysis of this new kind of datum we have found a new way of observing a link between the networks of meaning of the dream and of wakefulness. We observe this link not by focusing on the nature of the connection of specific contents of the networks noting the experiential similarity between the two. In the absence of some information regarding the nature of the network of meaning of the dream, such connections and similarities may be superficial and unrelated to the meanings that lie behind them. Rather, we observe the link between the networks of meaning of the dream and of wakefulness through the meaningfulness in which we experience the dream. That is, it is the way in which we experience the dream (i.e., meaningfully) that the connection between the networks come to the fore. We cannot observe the network of meaning that is present in the course of the dream. It remains hidden because in order to determine its nature we must be awake. But we can nevertheless observe that that network was operative and that it was closely related to the network of meaning of wakefulness. It is through the "experiential quality of meaningfulness" that is experienced in relation to the dream that we get to see the "halo," so to speak, of the earlier activation of the current network of meaning and that we come to know of the similarity between the networks.

The existence of the previously missing evidence of similarity of the networks of meaning of the dream and the awake individual, ultimately, allows us to apply to the dream the general assumptions underlying the psychoanalytic method, and thus to apply to the dream the psychoanalytic method with the conviction that the products of the application of this method will be discovered meaning. Meaning may be discovered in the dream through the application of the psychoanalytic method. This is what we sought to know. But we can say significantly more than this. The evidence of similarity emerges in such a way that not only may we discover the meaning of the dream, but we can discover meaning that is relevant to us as awake individuals. Were we to procure only evidence of the dream having intentions that were discernible by the awake analyzer, for example, we would be able to discover the meaning of the dream, but we could not know whether this meaning was telling us anything about ourselves. The network of meaning of the dream may be foreign to us. In contrast, the evidence of similarity of the networks allows us to know both of the presence of an intentional network of meaning during the dream and of its being related, and thus relevant, to that of the awake individual.

Upon finding that the general assumptions underlying psychoanalysis' method for the discovery of meaning may be applied to the dream and upon concluding that it is reasonable to contend that the application of this method to the dream will result in the discovery of meaning as it does when the method is applied to the individual's wakeful expressions, we have completed the Holistic justification of the psychoanalytic theory of the dream. It was not our aim to prove, nor have we proven—as Freud attempted to do in his *The Interpretation of Dreams* and as Grünbaum now demands of Freud—that the meanings that are arrived at through the application of the psychoanalytic method are true independently of the broader theoretical considerations that apply to the entire theory. We have clearly not shown, as Freud at points tried to, that the analysis of each single dream can provide a foundation for the entire dream theory. What we have shown is that the meanings that are discovered through the application of the psychoanalytic method to the dream are as true as are the meanings that are derived from the application of that method to our wakeful expressions; that the psychoanalytic theory of dreams is as valid as the broader edifice of psychoanalytic theory. This is quite a lot. Modern epistemology has taught us that to be respectably justified one may, and inevitably does, rely on the broader framework of thought within which one is working. One does not find anew the foundations of thought through the analysis of each particular instance. This is the basis of the Holistic approach to justification. Although this approach recognizes the influence of our theoretical constructions on how we perceive and formulate new domains, it is a far cry from the hermeneuticist approach that has emerged in psychoanalysis that maintains that in psychoanalysis there is no objective evidence because all is tainted by the subject's perspective and all theories are preferred narratives (chapter 1). The careful argumentation on the basis of detailed study of the evidence that went into the present study makes evident the fundamental difference between the approaches.

The bottom line here is that if one rejects the validity of the entire edifice of psychoanalytic theory, then one should also reject the psychoanalytic dream theory. However, if one considers the psychoanalytic theory to be well founded, then the dream theory should also be considered to be well founded. This is not because the dream theory has been proven independently of the broader theory, nor is it because of some arbitrary expansion of the theory in order to include a range of new assumptions that underlie the dream theory. Rather it is because the dream theory meshes well with the assumptions and networks of ideas that underlie the broader theory. This could have not been the case. The dream theory could have failed to interact well with the broader psychoanalytic theory. In fact, from our perspective it almost failed. We almost had to conclude that the psychoanalytic theory of dreams was without foundation. It was only through the delineation and explication of the specific nature of the "experiential quality of meaningfulness"—an experience previously neglected in the scientific literature—that psychoanalysis's general assumptions could be legitimately applied to the dream and the foundation for the theory found.

One Final Doubt: Can the Meaning of All Dreams be Discovered?

Can the meaning of *all* dreams be discovered? We have shown that the "experiential quality of meaningfulness" informs us of the similarity between the networks of meaning of the dream and of the awake individual. But may we assume that this similarity is pervasive? Is it not possible that this similarity is present only at those points in dreams that when we are awake arouse in us the "experiential quality of meaningfulness"? If similarity of the networks is limited in this way, what follows from this is that the possibility of discovering meaning in the dream is also limited. That is, what is suggested here is that there may be a limitation on discovering meaning in the dream, not determined by the skill of the analyst or the availability of information (e.g., associations), but rather by an inherent limitation on the very possibility of discovering meaning. Only the meaning of those fragments of dreams that arouse in us this experience could ever possibly be discovered. We must address this final doubt regarding the possibility of discovering meaning in the dream. The question is basically whether it is possible to generalize from the similarity that we know to exist at those points in the dream in relation to which we experience the "experiential quality of meaningfulness" when awake, to the network of meaning that is present at other parts of the dream, or more generally to other dreams.

My answer is as follows: It is possible to present a case for the generalizability of the similarity of the network of meaning. Such a case would be built on the following considerations:

a. There are many experiences regarding which we consider the momentary conscious experience to be an indicator of an underlying state that persists beyond the moments of the experience. For example, we consider the experience of mourning to reflect an underlying state of mourning that persists beyond the moments in which the experience is consciously felt. Even when the individual is feeling nothing, or feeling some other experience, we may ascribe to him or her the underlying state of mourning. Thus it is clearly *possible* that an experience would be an indicator of a state that persists beyond the momentary experience. Consequently, the state reflecting the similarity of the network of meaning of the dream with that of wakefulness may continue beyond the point regarding which it is expressed.

b. If we do not generalize regarding the similarity of the networks of meaning of the dream and of wakefulness beyond the point in relation to which the "experiential quality of meaningfulness" is felt, then we would have to conclude that the network of meaning during the dream is in a state of fluctuation. At points it is similar to that of the awake individual and at other points it is not. It is questionable whether the notion that during the dream there is a fluctuating network of meaning is a more reasonable hypothesis than the hypothesis that during the dream the network of meaning remains static. How, for example, would we explain these fluctuations? Especially within a single dream the notion of such fluctuations would be strange. If there are such fluctuations, we would expect that they would arouse feelings of surprise in the dreamer at those points in the dream in which the network of meaning that is active is similar to that of wakefulness. But this does not appear to be the case, at least as it emerges from the recall of dreams.

If the network remains static, we would have to assume that it remains the same as it is at the points in which we observe it to be similar to the network of meaning of the awake individual, because it is only at those points that we get to see its basic network of meaning.

c. It is my experience that in the course of the process of interpreting a dream there is an expansion of the "experiential quality of meaningfulness" in relation to it. The expansion of the experience suggests that a state reflecting the similarity between the networks of meaning of the dream and of the awake individual existed prior to its experience. This provides further support for the notion that even when the experience is absent, the state that it reflects is present. This support is, however, somewhat weak. This evidence from the clinical situation may be contaminated by the fact that in the course of the process of dream interpretation there is a focus on the understanding on the dream, and it is often the case that this understanding leads to a post hoc *recognition* of meaningfulness—that is, the recognition of there being apparently meaningful connections expressed in the dream. There would be value to this evidence of the expansion of the "experiential quality of meaningfulness" only if it is clearly distinguished from the recognition of the apparently meaningful connection. This is because, as we have seen, this recognition does not provide evidence of the continuity of the networks. Within the clinical situation it is not always possible to make such clear distinctions. In any case, more instances of such expansion of the "experiential quality of meaningfulness" within the clinical setting would have to be accumulated before a strong claim could be made on its basis.

While it is *possible* on the basis of these considerations to build a case in favor of the generalizability of the similarity of the networks of meaning of the dream and of wakeful life, in the final analysis, it must be admitted that the case is not airtight. Although it seems less likely that within a single dream the network of meaning that underlies it is shifting from one form to another, there remains the possibility that there are different kinds of dreams, some whose meaning may be discovered, others whose meaning may not. At the present state of research of the complex dimensions related to meaning and experience that I have set forth in this study, it would be best to avoid far-reaching generalizations. To conclusively determine whether indeed *all* dreams contain meaning that may be discovered through the application of the psychoanalytic method, we must await further examination.

THE "EXPERIENTIAL QUALITY OF MEANINGFULNESS" AS A UNIQUE FORM OF EXPERIENCE

As we come to the close of this chapter it may be wondered why the "experiential quality of meaningfulness" allowed for the Holistic justification of the psychoanalytic theory of dreams. Throughout this chapter we have seen *how* it does this. But on some "meta" level there is the question of why specifically this experience allowed for the justification. Is there something special in the essential nature of the experience that accounts for this fact? I believe that there is, and that it is worthwhile to bring this special feature to the fore.

In discussing the nature of the "experiential quality of meaningfulness" we recognized that this experience is a quality of our experiencing of meaning; it has an adverbial nature. It expresses an adverb (or quality) of experiencing (as in "experiencing x-ly"). In other words, by saying that we have the "experiential quality of meaningfulness" what we mean is that we are experiencing a connection meaningful*ly*. We saw how this allowed us to look at a dimension of the meaning connection other than that of content. But would any wakeful experience of an adverbial nature lead to the justification of the dream theory? Were one to experience the dream sadly, anxiously, humorously, and so on, would this provide us the necessary information regarding the continuity between the networks of meaning of the dream and of wakefulness? The examination of this question leads to an understanding of what is unique about the "experiential quality of meaningfulness."

If what we mean by experiencing sadly, anxiously, humorously, and so on, is that the awake individual experiences these feelings (e.g., sadness) when he or she passes the dream through his or her mind, then this form of experience does not provide evidence of similarity between the networks of meaning of the dream and of wakefulness. As we have seen in the course of this chapter, as well as in chapter 3, such experiences may be carryovers from the dream, or responses to the dream, which as such are not informative regarding the state or nature of the network of meaning of the dream. If, however, what we mean by experiencing the dream in these various experiential ways is that while awake we are experiencing that there is some meaning in the dream—albeit presently vague or unknown—that has something to do with sadness, with anxiety, or with humor, then the matter is different. This is because the vague experience that there is "something 'there' having to do with one of these feelings" is a composite experience comprised of these specific feelings, but also comprised of the "experiential quality of meaningfulness." It is the "experiential quality of meaningfulness" together with the experience that the meaningful connection is of a specific kind—that is, that it is tied to something sad, anxiety-arousing, funny, and so on. (e.g., the experience of sad meaningfulness). As such it is a subcategory of the "experiential quality of meaningfulness" and for the reasons already discussed this does allow us to know of the network of meaning that is present during the dream.

The "experiential quality of meaningfulness" emerges here as the most primary and abstract of experiences of connectedness between psychic entities. It is the very experience of the meaningful connectedness, without any further comment on the specific way in which the entities are connected. Other adverbial modifiers consist of the primary and abstract "experiential quality of meaningfulness" *plus* further characterization. But what informs us of the state of the network of meaning during the dream is only the pure "experiential quality of meaningfulness" dimension of the modifier.

We may conclude here that the "experiential quality of meaningfulness" is a quality of experiencing of meaning of the highest abstraction from the contents of the entities to which it refers. It is the most pure, abstract, content-free, expression of the connection between psychic entities that is possible. It is only a reflection of the statement that "something is connected to something." This accounts for its unique capacity to support the justification of the psychoanalytic dream theory. Through this particular experience, we see the workings of the network of meaning without requiring any direct substantive content of the network to be seen. Without presuppositions regarding the network of meaning from which they emerge, contents in themselves can tell us nothing. Regarding the dream, we are precluded from making such presuppositions by the inherent unobservability (to our wakeful network) of the network of meaning that may be present in its course. Thus it is only by transcending content, as we do through the "experiential quality of meaningfulness," that we can learn of the nature of the network. Through the abstractness of the connection expressed in this experiencing, we get to *see* the network, not directly, but through the "halo" that arises from its functioning. By being removed from content, rather than being immersed in it, the "experiential quality of meaningfulness" provides the most pure note of our presence.

CHAPTER SIX

Conclusions

There is a great deal of unmapped country within us which would have to be taken into account in an explanation of our gusts and storms.

— George Eliot, *Daniel Deronda*

*W*e have traversed a long and winding path from the first clarification of the issue of the possibility of discovering meaning in the dream in chapter 1, until the conclusions that we reached regarding this issue in chapter 5. Having arrived at our final destination, we may now take a look back and wonder what we have gained through this journey. And indeed, the path we took in the examination of the theoretical question addressed here should be likened to a journey, for, as in a journey, the value of the effort is not measured solely by what is attained at the end-point. Many valuable developments may emerge as one strives to that point.

In the present study, the end-point, the bottom line in and of itself, may seem not to have taken us far away from the point of departure. Adherents of psychoanalysis have widely accepted the psychoanalytic dream theory without adequate justification. Now we see that if one adheres to the broader framework of psychoanalysis, then the acceptance of the dream theory is justified. The step taken may seem to be small. However, when seen in the context of the entire journey, the breadth of this step may be recognized. In the following pages I will present the implications of this study within this broader context.

THE DREAM THEORY COULD HAVE FAILED

What we found in the present study is not the simple fact that the psychoanalytic theory of dreams is justified, but that clearly there was the possibility that it would have been found to be *un*justified. If the dream theory were found to be baseless, this would have far-reaching implications. Thus, the fact that it emerged that it does have a sound basis is also a very significant finding.

A NEW APPROACH TO THE JUSTIFICATION OF THEORIES WITHIN PSYCHOANALYSIS HAS BEEN FOUND TO BE BENEFICIAL

The attempts to justify psychoanalytic theories have traditionally vacillated between two basic, and often rival, forms: clinical case studies and empirical research. In the present study we have introduced another method, one that became necessary under the circumstances. It involved carrying out a critical rational analysis both of the theoretical framework of psychoanalysis and of certain kinds of experiences that may arise in the context of the dream, primarily the "experiential quality of meaningfulness." This approach highlighted the importance of attunement to experiential dimensions not only for therapeutic or analytic aims, but for the process of examination of theoretical propositions as well. It was also seen to be an approach that allows for the potential falsification or support of theoretical propositions, as well as for the critical examination of domains that are not readily amenable to simple empirical verification. As such, this approach emerges not only as an important alternative—at certain crucial points—to the clinical and empirical methods, but also as an alternative to the hermeneuticist position that has infiltrated psychoanalysis in recent years and has declared any form of justification obsolete. Thus, the methodological approach of this study may be usefully applied to the examination of other theoretical propositions, such as propositions regarding the nature of fantasies existing in the mind of the infant.

THE EXPLORATION OF FUNDAMENTAL ISSUES WITHIN PSYCHOANALYSIS ENRICHES THE THEORY

In order to explore the specific question of whether it is possible to discover the meanings of dreams through the application of the psychoanalytic method, it became necessary to formulate and reformulate some of the foundations of the psychoanalytic theory. Even to understand *how come* there is a question, we had to go to the heart of psychoanalytic thinking. There are many reasons why Freud's dream theory was not seriously questioned by generations of analysts. But among these reasons is the fact that the way in which the theory is often presented does not allow the question to be seen. It is taken for granted that the dream, like any other psychic product, has meaning. It is only when we delved into the issues of the meaning of meaning in psychoanalysis and of what makes a certain psychic product a meaningful one, that the question in relation to the dream came to the surface. The result of this was that in examining whether the meaning of the dream can be discovered the framework of the psychoanalytic theory was enriched. Tracing our steps, the following formulations may be considered most significant.

The Formulation of the Concept of Meaning within Psychoanalysis and Its Distinction from Other Kinds of Meanings

When we first raised the question of whether meaning can be discovered it became necessary to define what we mean by "meaning" and by the "*discovery* of meaning." We delineated the different forms of meaning—that is, meaning to the observer versus meaning within the subject, and meaning of stating versus meaning of the statement. Focusing on the meaning of the statement, we further distinguished between three categories—meaning created, meaning described, and meaning discovered—and highlighted the importance of the distinction between them. We particularly emphasized that there is value in distinguishing between meaning discovered—that is, meaning as an actual causal connection between psychic entities within the individual's network of meaning—and the other categories of meaning that are not concerned with the actuality of the connection, but rather with thematic and subjective ties that may be found between the entities. In recent years, with the growing popularity of the psychoanalytical hermeneuticist approach, the nature of this distinction has been blurred. The result has been the creation of a false opposition between "meaning" and actual causal events and consequently confusion regarding the possibility of attaining the psychoanalytic goal of coming in touch with one's actual personal truth. Thus, our clarification of the issue of meaning not only created space for the study of the issue of the possibility of discovering meaning in the dream, but in a more general way created a space for psychoanalysis to continue with its pursuit of truth as actual causal events existing within the individual.

The Formulation of the Nature of Justification within Psychoanalysis in the Light of Developments in the Field of Epistemology

The question we asked regarding the possibility of discovering the meaning of the dream is an epistemological one. To answer the question it became necessary to explore the different forms of justification that epistemology has to offer. It became apparent that psychoanalytic propositions were being evaluated, both by Freud and his followers and by his critics, according to criteria derived from Atomistic forms of justification. Holistic forms of justification, widely accepted within contemporary epistemology, were not adequately integrated. In the present study we integrated this form of justification. The psychoanalytic dream theory was measured by the degree to which it fits into the broader network of psychoanalytic ideas. The exploration of the issue of justification within psychoanalysis and the ultimate integration of the Holistic approach not only contributed to answering the question of this study. It also provides a basis for the future exploration of other psychoanalytic propositions and points to the fact that it is important for psychoanalysis to maintain a dialogue with other disciplines. As we have seen through the present study, such interchange makes obsolete the sometimes-heard psychoanalytic claim that psychoanalysis is so unique that it cannot be subject to any form of critical study acceptable to other scientific disciplines. Indeed, if the complexity of other fields is recognized—in our case the complexity of the philosophical field of epistemology—then it may be seen that psychoanalytic formulations may be carefully studied while their unique nature is carefully taken into account.

The Formulation of a Psychoanalytic Model of Meaning and Its Discovery and the Exploration of Some of Its Underlying Assumptions

To examine whether the psychoanalytic dream theory could be Holistically justified, it became necessary to formulate some of the major basic assumptions underlying the general psychoanalytic theory of discovery of meaning. In turn, the formulation of these assumptions required the formulation of a model of the mind that is implicit in psychoanalysis. This model centered on the mind as a container of the individual's meanings. In bringing this model to light, we dealt with some of the limitations of Freud's topographical and structural models as well as contemporary models, which focus on the integration of meaning into the self. We differentiated between integrated and split-off meanings, which are distinguished by the degree to which the psychic entities involved are in a interconnected "knowing" or "aboutness" causal relationship, as opposed to a "blind" causal relationship. On the basis of this model we proceeded to delineate the three basic assumptions: the assumption of effective and rational communication of intentions, the assumption of original connectedness, and the assumption of cross-temporal accessibility.

The implications of the psychoanalytic model of meaning and the related assumptions underlying the discovery of meaning could not be elaborated in the present study beyond the discussion of the issues that specifically related to the possibility of discovering meaning in the dream. It is clear, however, that the model and the assumptions contribute to the understanding of the foundations of psychoanalytic thought. Moreover, the fact that in this study the evidential basis and support of the assumptions were explicated allows for critical evaluation of the foundations, rather than merely a presentation of them.

Clarification of the Basic Propositions of the Freudian Dream Theory

Our extensive analysis of Freud's dream theory in the light of our clarification of the term *meaning* allowed us to see that Freud's proposition regarding meaning in the dream was comprised of two basic propositions (chapter 2). The first proposition was that the dream is a meaningful statement. By this Freud meant that the dream contains underlying unconscious intentions (e.g., "I really did mean that my friend R. was a simpleton—like my Uncle Josef"[Freud, 1900, p. 139]). The second proposition was that the meanings of all dreams are wishes. Here Freud was referring to the nature of psychic force that motivates the dreams (e.g., the psychic force behind the dream that R. was a simpleton was the wish to receive the title professor). The proposition that the dream is meaningful and the proposition that the meaning of the dream is a wish were seen to refer to the meaning of the statement and the meaning of stating, respectively.

One consequence of the distinction between these two different kinds of propositions was that the proposition regarding the wishful nature of the dream was seen to assume a secondary role and not to be inherent to Freud's more central and essential proposition regarding the dream's very meaningfulness. The former proposition would arise only when one would inquire into the question of *why* the meaningful statements in the dream are being made, and could be discarded without affecting the more basic latter one.

This clarification contributes to the understanding of a fundamental aspect of Freud's thought and its relationship to contemporary dream theory. Freud's great discovery was that meaningful statements contained in the dream could be revealed by applying the psychoanalytic method, not that underlying these statements were wishes. Consequently all the innovations that point to the unwishful origin of the dream or to other psychic forces that motivate it can no longer be considered dismissive of Freudian dream theory. As long as they are accompanied by a concern with the meanings that are expressed in the dream these innovations must be seen rather to be elaborations of Freud's most essential claim regarding the dream. Recognizing the tie between Freudian thought and contemporary psychoanalysis is important in order to understand and assess the foundations of our current clinical and theoretical formulations and also to avoid unnecessary dissent and schism that has often been harmful to the development of the psychoanalysis (Blass & Simon, 1994).

Clarification of the Affective-Experiential Approach within Psychoanalysis

In the course of our examination of recent developments in the psychoanalytic theory of dreams we distinguished between the classical Ideational-Textual approach to meaning and the more recent Affective-Experiential approach. The latter approach—emerging mainly in the writings of Winnicott and Bion and their disciples—placed a special emphasis on meaning as an experiential event. However, what this means exactly was left quite obscure and at times mystical. Our analysis of this approach in the light of the psychoanalytic model of meaning that we had formulated allowed for the clarification of the obscurities. It became possible to see how the Affective-Experientialists were speaking of the integration of meaning through the full experience of one's experience, that in the full experience of one's experiences the interconnections between psychic entities are revived. It was then also possible to see the nature of the relationship between the Affective-Experiential approach and the classical Ideational-Textual one. The latter approach was also seen to be concerned with experience, but with the experience of the connection between the psychic entities. That is, it is the experience of the connection that leads to integration. The two approaches basically agree on the meaning of meaning, but differ regarding the means of integrating it.

This clarification is important not only to the understanding of the possibilities of justifying the psychoanalytic theory of dreams. Nor is its additional value only in furthering our understanding of yet another psychoanalytic approach. Rather its special value is derived from the fact that it allows for the understanding of an important experiential path to the integration of meaning. As a clear and reasonable theoretical formulation, rather than one that is shrouded in obscurity, it may be incorporated with the broader psychoanalytic theory. In this way psychoanalysis can do away with mystical propositions that are inappropriate in this realm and avoid false schisms between classical and experiential approaches.

An Understanding of the "Experiential Quality of Meaningfulness" and the Path It Opens to the Understanding of Other Experiences

The justification of the psychoanalytic theory of the dream ultimately emerged through the analysis of the meaning of the "experiential quality of meaningfulness." This analysis was based on a critical rational analysis of the special phenomenological characteristics of this experiential quality and provided a deep understanding of the intrapsychic state that it reflects. As such, this analysis may be seen to contribute to the theory of affects in two major ways. It both clarifies the meaning of an experience that had never before been the subject of study, and provides a framework for the analysis of other experiences.

In sum, the theoretical yield of this study is considerable. But the yield is not only in the realm of theory.

CLINICAL IMPLICATIONS

Although the end-product of this study is the support of the psychoanalytic method in the context of the dream, the process through which the support is attained and what emerged in its course point to the fact that the study also has some very important implications for the clinical situation. These may be divided into two major groups: general implications for the clinical situation and implications in terms of dream analysis. It is in the latter that we come to a surprising conclusion regarding the value of the dream interpretation.

The General Clinical Implication: Attunement to the "Experiential Quality of Meaningfulness"

This study has shown that the "experiential quality of meaningfulness" indicates the presence of the activation of a meaningful connection. As such, the attunement to this experience, not only in relation to the dream, but within the broader clinical setting, is of importance. When the patient reports that he or she experiences meaningfulness it should be taken as an actual sign of the presence of something meaningful. This may seem at first to be the intuitive response to such a report, yet as we have seen there are the possibilities that one would relate to it as a report of an illusory experience or an additional dimension of the content (or the script) that is being expressed, and not as a source of veridical evidence regarding the presence of such a meaningful activation of connections within the network of meaning. That is, one may mistakenly consider such a report to be an expression of the individual's misguided belief that there is something meaningful taking place, or that through the expression of this experience the individual is saying something regarding the content of which he or she is speaking. For example, if the patient were to report an "experiential quality of meaningfulness" in relation to an encounter with her boss, it may be suggested that the experience is derived from a wish to experience something meaningful in relation to this boss, or that the meaning of meaningfulness to this patient is love, or fear, or some other kind of feeling or idea, and that she is actually expressing these other feelings and ideas through the experience. The present study dispels these alternative possibilities. If what is being expressed is indeed an "experiential quality of meaningfulness," and not a belief that there is a meaningful tie present based on the assessment of the contents, then the experience provides veridical evidence regarding the activation of a meaningful connection.

Of course, for the report of an "experiential quality of meaningfulness" to be of value, it would have to be clearly distinguished from reports of the "experiential quality of meaningfulness" that emerge solely from the assessment of the contents. This distinction, while apparent at certain times, especially introspectively, may at other times be difficult to make. The attunement to the "experience of meaningfulness" would require careful listening to this fine, yet very significant, distinction.

Clinical Implications in Terms of Dream Analysis: Dream Interpretations as a Possible "Royal Road"

This study has several important clinical implications for the way in which one should relate to the dream within the clinical setting. First, *the present study has pointed to the importance of distinguishing in the context of dream interpretation between discovered meanings and other categories of meaning* (i.e., created and described meanings). We have shown that the network of meaning of the awake analyzer is similar to that of the dreamer, but there remains the possibility that in the clinical situation the patient will not actualize this similarity. That is, our study has shown that similarity exists, that it is *possible* to touch the network of the dream, that wakeful associations *can* connect to what is being expressed in the dream, but in practice there is also the possibility that the patient will *not* connect, will *not* associate in a way that will allow the patient entrance into the dream; that despite the actual link of the dream to the wakeful network, in practice the dream will remain a foreign stimuli, like a Rorschach inkblot, to which the associations are merely elaborations of the familiar analyzing network of meaning. Indeed we may learn about the individual through such elaborations, through the analysis of the meanings she assigns to her dreams, and through the analysis of what she believes to be the meanings of her dream. But it is necessary to distinguish between the understanding that emerges from such analyses and the meanings that actually exist in the dream. We must thus wonder whether the associations that the patient is offering are really touching the network of meaning that was underlying the dream.

Such detachment from the network of what is being expressed may occur in other situations as well. Despite what we have seen to be the actual continuity between our present network of meaning and those of the past, in practice, our associations to events of the past may not link us to the network of the past, but rather only to our current one. This will allow us a deeper understanding of how we presently consider our past, but it will not lead us to a deeper understanding of our past, to the meanings that we actually expressed then. If the meanings of the past are actually influencing our present state, if it is important for us to actually know our personal truth, then it is important to recognize the meanings of the past and not only our present conceptions of them. In this case there would be value to being aware of when the analyzing network is relating from a detached stance to the expressing network and when it is relating from a linked stance. The same can be said of the dream. *If the meanings in the dream are actually influencing us, if we wish to know the truth about what is being expressed in the dream, then we must distinguish between the meanings we presently assign to the dream and the meanings that are actually expressed in it.*

This leads us to our next point. Does the dream indeed provide us with meanings that extend beyond the scope of what is regularly available to the analyzing network of meaning? That is, is there any point in making the special effort to understand the meanings that were expressed at the time of the dream? Do they differ in any way from the meanings that could have been expressed by a current wakeful network? Are dreams not simply expressions identical to those of wakefulness, just somewhat more complexly packaged and hence more difficult to understand? If this were the case, there would be no point to struggle to attain their meaning. Unlike the meaning of the past event, the meaning of the dream would be no different from other meanings that would be accessible from analysis of current wakeful expressions. Here we enter the heated debate regarding the question of whether the dream is a special source of meaning. Should the dream deserve a special status as a context that allows for greater access to more deeply hidden meanings and/or to meanings not as readily available through the analysis of wakeful material?

In the course of the present study what we have managed to show thus far was that the dream allows for access to some meaning. This in itself took considerable effort. We have not dealt with the question of whether it allows for access to any especially earlier, deeper, or more repressed meanings. We have not shown that the analysis of the dream opens the path to meanings that could not be just as readily derived from the analysis of our present wakeful statements. Further analysis, however, reveals that this study does indeed provide some support for the notion that the dream actually does allow for this. This possibility arises from the fact that, as we have seen, during dreams there is a state in which meanings are being expressed even though the contents through which they find expression do not provide any apparent clue to the nature of the meanings. It may be the case that in wakefulness there is often no immediate connection between the contents expressed and the meanings that underlie them. But the immediate contents draw our attention and we make judgments concerning these contents based on our ideas and beliefs about ourselves and the world. We see connections between contents in part because we have ideas regarding how things are connected. The lack of such *apparent* connections in the dream provides a greater opportunity to experience the meaningfulness of meanings regarding which we know nothing in terms of the content. There may be a greater possibility of feeling for the first time the very existence of meanings that are completely unknown to us. As such the dream constitutes a special context not only in terms of the problematic unobservability of the network of meaning that is present in its course, but also in terms of the meanings to which it allows accessibility. *Not only is it possible to discover the meaning of dreams, but it is possible to discover meanings that could not be as readily accessed through the analysis of our wakeful expressions.*

This conclusion supports the view that it is indeed important in the context of dream interpretation to distinguish between meanings that are discovered and those that arise in relation to the dream, but are not contained in it. If we are to come to recognize those meanings that lie beyond what is available to us while we are awake, then we must strive to discover the meanings that actually are being expressed in the dream. Technical developments follow from this. For example, an additional focus in the clinical setting should be placed on facilitating the patient's becoming linked to his or her dream, and clinical attunement should be directed toward discerning between associations that come from within the mind of the dreamer and those that come from the more remote stance of the detached wakeful observer. The details of the technical developments that become necessary in the light of these findings remain to be carefully worked out, but an important first step in this direction is the very awareness of the possibility that from the analysis of dreams there may emerge meaning in very different kinds of senses of the term.

A further implication of this study for dream analysis has to do with the fact that the dream is a special context not only in terms of the discovery of meaning. It is also a special context of experience. The Affective-Experiential approach has emphasized this. It has spoken of the dream as a unique area of play, as a space for new experiences, as a phenomenon to be experienced rather than understood, and so on. But this approach has not provided an adequate explanation of the dream's experiential uniqueness. The present study does provide a basis for an explanation of this uniqueness. To recall, from the perspective of the Affective-Experiential approach, it is when contents are fully experienced that the underlying ideational connections within the network of meaning are actualized. In the course of this study we have justified the notion that what is being actualized through the experience of the dream are indeed real connections within the network of meaning. It may now be seen that the absence of *apparently* meaningful connections within the contents of the dream provides a special opportunity for the full experience of the contents (and hence a special opportunity for actualization). As in the case of the special access to deeply hidden meanings that the dream facilitates, what underlies the dream's special capacity to facilitate important experiential events is the lack of interference from our thoughts and beliefs regarding the connections between the contents.

It should be emphasized, however, that what is facilitated in terms of experience is not only the powerful and free experience of contents, but the "experiential quality of meaningfulness" itself. Beyond the scope of the experiences that are of interest from the perspective of the affective-experiential approach there is the "experiential quality of meaningfulness" that finds its most pure expression in the absence of the apparent connections between contents. That is, the dream provides a special context in which the individual becomes integrated through the full experience of the dream contents, but in which she also comes to recognize herself as an integrated network of meaning through the direct and immediate experiential knowledge of the presence of her network of meaning.

Here too, the question of how to translate these findings regarding the dream into practice remains an open issue. It would seem, however, that one direction would be a greater awareness to the ways in which the patient uses dreams and relates to them. For example, it may be the case that indeed for certain patients the full and close experience of the dream would indeed be more important than any understanding of it. This may be true for individuals whose thought has become detached from experience or has become overly directive and forced. For these people the freedom from interfering thoughts that the dream allows for may be particularly valuable. Awareness to the ways in which the patient uses her dreams would be in line with the Affective-Experiential approach with two differences: (1) alongside other experiences there would be a focus on the "experiential quality of meaningfulness," and (2) the involvement with the special experiential dimensions of the dream would not imply the adoption of a semimystical stance in relation to it. It would now be possible to understand these special dimensions in terms of the processes that are taking place within the network of meaning.

One further implication of this study for the analysis of dreams in the clinical context remains to be discussed. This last implication has to do with the fact that there still remains the question of whether *all* dreams have discoverable meaning. In the course of this study we saw that what ultimately allowed for the justification of the psychoanalytic dream theory was the similarity that was shown to exist between the network of meaning of the dream and that of wakefulness. What remained inconclusively answered was the extent to which this similarity could be generalized beyond the specific situations in which the "experiential quality of meaningfulness" was present, to situations in which no such experience was felt. That is, there remained the possibility that there is not always similarity between the networks. It seemed quite likely that when the networks within a certain dream were at a specific moment seen to be similar, then the networks were similar throughout the dream. And a good case was made for the similarity of the networks of the dream and of wakefulness in *all* dreams. Nevertheless, there remained the possibility that the networks of meaning of dreams that revealed no indications of similarity (through the "experiential quality of meaningfulness"), indeed were not similar to the networks of meaning of wakefulness. The conclusion was that we cannot know for sure that all dreams are amenable to having their meaning discovered through the application of the psychoanalytic method. *There may be dreams whose meaning we cannot discover.* While it may be that many dreams are brought to analysis because of the feeling of meaningfulness that emerges in relation to them, it also may be the case that there are dreams that are reported without any such immediate experience, whose meanings are not accessible to us and regarding which we cannot even know whether they contain meaning.

One consequence of this should be a certain openness within the clinical situation to the possibility that not *all* dreams have meaning. The translation of this consequence into practice would be complex. It would involve adopting a somewhat different attitude toward the dream. For example, we would have to leave room for wondering whether getting stuck in the understanding of a certain dream is informative of the meaning of the dream, or informative of the fact that the dream has no meaning, or at least none that is accessible to the wakeful analyzer. We would have to simultaneously pursue the hidden meanings behind the possible defensive maneuvers of the dream and ask ourselves whether there are any meanings there. The meanings that we do arrive at in the course of the interpretative process would also have to be more carefully scrutinized: Are these meanings indeed *discovered* meanings?

The openness to the possibility that there are dreams whose meanings are not available to us may also imply that greater attention should be paid to those dreams in which the "experiential quality of meaningfulness" is more pronounced. For in those dreams we have greater assurance that indeed the meanings that are uncovered in the course of the interpretative process are meanings that are indeed *discovered* and not meanings that are "formed" by the awake analyzer.

The conclusions of this study regarding dream analysis may be somewhat surprising. Throughout we have seen how very difficult it was to demonstrate that the dream has accessible meaning whatsoever. Having found that it does, the dream ultimately emerges as a context that allows for *special* access to meaning, both experientially and in terms of recognizing the specific connections that underlie the experiences. But from another angle it becomes apparent that this "royal road" to the unconscious is not without pitfalls. There is the danger that *in practice* instead of discovering meanings that actually exist within the dream we will only assign to the dream new meanings that emerge from our wakeful reaction to it. Furthermore, we have not succeeded in completely doing away with the possibility that regarding some dreams all that can be done is assign new meanings; that for some there may be no way of discovering their meaning or even of knowing that they have any meaning at all. Under these special conditions it would seem that the optimal clinical stance in the course of dream analysis would involve the combination of the psychoanalytic relentless pursuit of the various kinds of meanings that actually exist within the individual, together with a careful and limited doubt regarding the meaningfulness of some dreams. Such a stance would allow us to plummet the depths of the meanings of the dream and at the same time open a path to the future resolution of the question of whether indeed all dreams have discoverable meaning.

CONCLUSION

In 1900, Freud wrote that "the interpretation of dreams is the royal road to the knowledge of the unconscious activities of the mind" (Freud, 1900, p. 608). Although this statement is commonly taken to mean that dream analysis provides the best access to the individual's unconscious meanings, a careful reading of the context reveals that its more immediate meaning is that dream interpretation offers the best access to the understanding of the general processes of the mind. The continuation of the statement is as follows: "By analyzing dreams we can take a step forward in our understanding of the composition of that most marvelous and most mysterious of instruments. Only a small step, no doubt; but a beginning" (ibid.). Freud was speaking here of the value of dream interpretation to the understanding of broader mental processes.

The present study has furthered Freud's endeavor to stride toward a deeper understanding of the marvels and mysteries of the mind. Our path was not that of dream interpretation per se, but of a careful scrutiny of the theoretical framework that must underlie it and a careful exploration of the experiential dimensions with which it is involved. This path provided the necessary basic justification of the psychoanalytic theory of dreams. Relying on a Holistic model of justification, we showed that meanings can indeed be discovered through the application of the psychoanalytic method. But, as we have now seen, much more has been gained than this final important end-product. The journey along this path has proven very beneficial methodologically, theoretically, and ultimately clinically. New ways of justifying psychoanalytic propositions have been set forth, the foundations of the theory have been enriched, and implications for dream interpretation as well as the process of understanding other expressions within the clinical setting have been outlined.

Throughout this study I have tried to maintain a critical stance, rationally scrutinizing the data and the arguments, doubting basic psychoanalytic precepts, rather than accepting them on authority or tradition. At the same time, I have tried to remain as close and true as possible to experiential qualities of which I have come to know through careful analytic attunement to others as well as to myself. Some of these qualities were at times elusive and resistant to definition. I believe that I have shown that this critical and yet experientially near approach is possible and fruitful, and I hope that it will find application in the future research of psychoanalytic propositions. Such research—theoretical, clinical, and empirical—is needed in the field of dream theory in order to further substantiate and delimit the boundaries of the present study. Are *all* dreams indeed meaningful? Does systematically collected evidence support our claims regarding the meaning and value of the "experiential quality of meaningfulness"? I look forward with anticipation to these further steps toward "our understanding of the composition of that most marvelous and most mysterious of instruments."

NOTES

CHAPTER 1. THE CONTEXT

1. This will include, however, aspects of the writings of the philosophical hermeneuticist Ricouer on psychoanalysis because these have been so deeply incorporated into psychoanalytic hermeneuticism. My focus will be on how these writings have been regarded from within this latter perspective, rather than on a broader understanding of Ricouer's thinking, which, arguably, puts this perspective in question.

2. It should be noted that not all psychoanalytic hermeneuticists specifically refer to themselves as such, or characterize their work by the use of the term "hermeneutical" per se.

3. Renik is an exception in this regard. At times, he seems to be saying that his view of the inaccessibility of psychoanalytic facts is part of his broader view of the inaccessibility of objective facts in general (e.g., Renik, 1998, p. 491).

4. My exposition of the term meaning is not comprehensive and one should not wrongly conclude here that "meaning" refers *only* to relationships between concepts or between psychic events. For example, when we speak of certain kinds of metaphysical relationships physical entities may be involved as well (Danielou, 1957, p. 22; Tillich, 1957, p. 42).

5. Note that in these examples the focus is on psychic events and the question of whether or not they correspond to something that actually occurred in the external reality is totally irrelevant for our purposes. This dimension in no way detracts from the reality and concreteness of the event.

6. I am not speaking here of the tendency of some people to consider all their conceptions of the past as events that actually took place in external reality. Although it is difficult to accept that our meanings do not refer to real causal connections, the notion that the contents of our mind may be fantasy, not reflections of events that actually took place in external reality, can be readily incorporated.

7. It should be recalled that I am here speaking of hermeneuticism as it emerges within psychoanalysis. I am not referring to the more intricate models of hermeneuticism that have been developed outside of this field.

8. For a more comprehensive understanding of these basic epistemological terms see Dancy (1985).

9. Properly speaking, a theory is based on propositions, not pure data. Here, however, for the sake of simplicity, I define data as propositions about findings in observations, and thus I speak of data as a foundation.

10. There are various alternative proposals concerning how a theoretical proposition is to be based on observations. Primary among them are the methods of deduction and bootstrapping. According to the deductive method, evidence confirms a theoretical proposition if evidence can be appropriately deduced from it. The bootstrap method holds that a theoretical proposition is justified if it, or positive instances of it, can be deduced from observational propositions.

11. In mentioning the term "reality" I repeatedly emphasize "internal or external" as a reminder, in particular to the psychoanalytic reader, that "reality" is not to be taken as a reference specifically to events that actually occurred in the external world. Having a fantasy is also a reality.

12. There have been several attempts to look more systematically at Freud's use of the term meaning (e.g., Edelson, 1972, 1988; Foulkes, 1985; Peterfreund, 1971), the most detailed of these attempts being that of Shope (1973). These attempts explain Freud's use of the term through various categories, which allow for clarification in relation to several important dimensions (e.g., Freud's conception of symbols). But for the purpose of understanding Freud's position in relation to the meaning of the dream and its justification I consider the categories of meaning that I have proposed to be the most appropriate ones. Thus I will proceed to examine Freud's use of the term meaning in their light rather than lead the reader astray through explorations of the intricate relationships between my formulations and those of other writers.

13. The different senses of meaning may be seen to be embedded in Freud's statement that "By 'sense' we understand 'meaning', 'intention', 'purpose' and 'position in a continuous psychical context'" (1916a, p. 61).

14. The present section is based on a recent paper of mine in which I also discuss the clinical implications of such critical studies (Blass, 2001).

15. Welsh himself does not fill the absence to which he points. His book provides only a *literary* critical analysis of Freud.

16. It is perhaps strange that one of the more careful examinations of the justification of Freud's dream theory comes from Spence, who has been cited here as a representative figure of the hermeneutic approach to psychoanalysis. But then perhaps the failure to justify Freud's theories in accordance with the overly rigorous conditions that, as we will soon see, Spence requires could account for his later turn to hermeneuticism.

CHAPTER 2. FREUD'S JUSTIFICATION OF HIS DREAM THEORY

1. McLeod (1992) is an exception here. He has argued that this book contains merely the kernel of a truth that was later changed in the course of Freud's many revisions of his theory over the years. His arguments, however, are weak, especially relative to those of the consensual position that emphasizes the central position held by *The Interpretation of Dreams*.

2. It may, however, be the case that if the interpretative process ultimately failed to yield a coherent and intelligible comprehensive meaning, Freud would have conceded

that his specific steps were incorrect. Other complex interrelationships between the two routes may be found. However, the study of them would take us too far afield. It should also be noted at this point that ascribing to Freud these two routes of justification involves a benevolent reading of Freud's project. Explicit references to his actual procedure of justification involved are sorely absent in Freud's argument.

3. Here once again we may see the place of the literature review. If, as Freud misguidedly concluded from his summary of the literature, we may regard as fact that everything in the dream is derived from experience and that the dream is a transformation of ideas (see p. 73–74), then indeed there would be some preliminary basis for Freud's present contentions regarding the causal and meaningful connections between the dream and the events of wakefulness.

4. Later Freud would speak of different ways of fragmenting the dream (esp. Freud, 1923c, p. 109), but then too, the question remains unresolved as to why any one of the specific methods he mentions should yield fragments that, especially in relation to them, the associations which they arouse point to a relevant underlying thought.

5. In chapter 3, the great obstacles to assuming that the dream contains sensible and realistic statements will be discussed at length.

CHAPTER 3. CAN THE APPLICATION OF PSYCHOANALYTIC PRINCIPLES TO THE DREAM BE JUSTIFIED?

1. I use these terms for the sake of brevity. To be exact, the meaning does not reside in the entities themselves, but rather in the relationships between them.

2. In pragmatics there is a similar underlying assumption. Grice (1975, 1978), a major figure in that field, relies on this pragmatic assumption in his application of his "Principle of Cooperation" and the four "Maxims" that he deduces from them. Grice puts forth the view that, in contrast to the process that takes place in determining the semantic meaning of what is said, apparent deviations from effective and rational discourse should be taken as a form of expressing indirect meanings. Psychoanalysis, however, as we will see, takes this assumption further and focuses on the personal motivational, rather than conventional meanings.

3. Of course many other forms of intervention may take place at such a point. But my focus here is solely on the expansion of the text to make it appropriate for the discovery of meaning.

4. Of course one could create meaning—forge new links with a totally foreign or implanted psychic entity. This, however, would not lead to the discovery of meaning, our concern in the present context.

5. It may be noted that this assumption has an important implication that extends beyond the immediate issue of the possibility of discovering meaning. This pertains to the possibility of integration of the split-off meanings that we discover. Only if there had been an initial tie between the split-off entity and the integrated network of meanings would it be possible—by relating to the ties that we discern—for the split-off meaning to find its place within the network of meaning. By attending to the laughter that emerged in the course of telling a sad story, we may discover a split-off meaning (e.g., that hurting another means pleasure), but now this additional meaning must be *integrated*; it must find its place within the network of meaning. This integration is possible through the further elaboration of the connection between the laughter and its

source and the sadness and its source only if we assume the assumption of original connectedness. Given this assumption, the elaboration may be seen to revive the path
between the split-off meaning and the network, revive the mutual "knowing" relationship that has been lost. In the absence of this kind of original connectedness we would
not be able to integrate real ties that we discover into the network of meaning. We would
recognize meanings, but they would remain foreign.

      6. The implications of this assumption, like its predecessor, extend beyond dis-
covery of meaning to the issue of integration. If we do not assume a certain form of
cross-temporal accessibility, then it would not be possible to integrate into our present
network of meaning the meanings discovered in the past. The meanings would remain
foreign to our present selves.

      7. For further examples, one may return to some of the examples in chapter 1 in
the context of the meaning of discovering meaning in psychoanalysis.

      8. It will be apparent here that I do not consider motivational states that are not
determined by a network of meaning to be intentional states (e.g., motives emerging as a
result of organic disease). It will also be apparent that I consider all expressions of a network of meaning to be guided by intentions. If for some reason the network of meaning
started to randomly fire, the expressions would no longer be considered expressions of
that network of meaning. It is only when the network retains its integrity that it is possible to regard it as a network. Further elaboration of these points is beyond the scope of
the present study.

      9. I stress here "natural" in contrast to the situation in which coherence is espe-
cially sought out in relation to a text that is originally felt to be incoherent. Since to
some extent coherence can always be found, the latter situation would not be able to
serve as evidence.

      10. This problem does not arise regarding the first assumption when it is applied
to the wakeful situation because when the question of the existence of intentions arises
in that context, the two possible answers are either that intentions exist or that they do
not. There is no room for the possibility that perhaps intentions unrelated to the
person's wakeful network of meaning are being operated. If there are intentions that are
activated during the individual's *wakeful* state, then, trivially, they are related to the
person's *wakeful* network of meaning. In contrast, it is not immediately apparent that if
there are intentions that are activated during the individual's *dreaming* state that they
are related to the person's *wakeful* network of meaning. It may be obvious that these
latter intentions are related to the individual's dreaming network of meaning (if there is
one), but it would remain to be shown that they are related to the network of meaning
of the awake individual.

      11. One may wonder whether the experience of interpreting one's dream in the
course of the dream would not contradict this claim. However, if that interpretation is
considered to take place in the course of the dream, then it would also have to be considered part of the dream and as such interpretable in some state beyond the dream.
This points to the difficulty in singling out (from the perspective of the awake individual) any observing network of meaning that may be operative during the dream from
the dream itself. So even were the dreamer to begin to raise associations to his dream in
the course of his dream (although I have never heard of such a case), we would not be
able to determine that this is indeed an interpretative process and not a dream whose

manifest content is the interpretation of a dream, and about whose underlying meaning we know nothing.

12. We have seen how in wakefulness there is reason to believe that continuity exists between present and past networks. This is the nature of the accessibility between the two. In wakefulness, however, continuity is not *necessary*. It only becomes necessary when the network referred to is in no way available to us an object of study.

13. One may object that also in fantasizing we may find ourselves expressing attitudes similarly discordant with our general attitudes. However, the fantasy does not encompass the entire expression of our network of meaning. While we are maintaining a fantasy of desiring vanilla ice cream, we may still maintain our basic attitude of dislike for that flavor. In the dream we do not have such evidence of the retention of our basic attitudes.

14. Here too one should take into account that usually during a fantasy that occurs in wakefulness other processes are taking place simultaneously with the fantasizing; one's entire network of meaning is not centered on the fantasy. There are, for example, some observing processes going on as well. Regarding the dream, in contrast, we have no knowledge of additional processes and it appears that the entire network of meaning is centered on the dreaming. Consequently, we must conclude that in contrast to the wakeful fantasizing state, regarding the dream state we must conclude that if the content expressed therein is not having an impact on the wakeful network of meaning, then there is no impact whatsoever of the network of meaning during the dream on the wakeful network.

15. In a recent work the Israeli philosopher Oded Balaban (1995) in fact argues in favor of the claim that a network of meaning unrelated to that of wakefulness may be shown to be present in the course of the dream. According to him, the dream is expressive of intentions. His evidence rests on factors such as the absence of surprise over the strange events that occur in the course of the dream. It is only upon awakening that the events seem surprising. While the demonstration of the existence of a network of meaning in the dream would not contradict my present remarks regarding the problems with discerning intentions in practice, it should be noted that Balaban's argument in itself does not suffice to demonstrate the network's existence. Balaban overlooks the fact that our interpretation of the meaning of the feeling of surprise and the absence of it are based on an application of our regular wakeful network of meaning. Given the alternate network of meaning, the meaning of the absence of surprise may mean something completely different.

16. In fact, under such circumstances our associations to the dream would be even less informative than our associations to a Rorschach card. In the latter instance the nature of the stimulus is available to us. The situation in the dream would be more like association to an inkblot that no one else has seen.

Chapter 4. Developments Regarding the Dream Theory

1. The issue of Freud's retraction of his idea of the binding aim of the dream is beyond the scope of the present paper (Blass,1993).

2. One source of confusion in determining the essence of the Affective-Experiential approach is the fact that while the adherents of this approach often speak of expe-

riencing as an actualization of meaning, at other times they juxtapose "meaning" and "experiencing" (e.g., Pontalis, 1981, p. 33). An examination of the broader context reveals, however, that in the latter cases they are not juxtaposing meaning in general, but only meaning in the sense of a verbal understanding of the connections between psychic entities.

3. This enabling of experiencing is often considered an early developmental step and task. At some early preverbal stage, integration of meaning requires some form of containment of experience. But my present exposition points to the ongoing role of this containment and experiencing in the attempt to integrate meaning.

CHAPTER 5. THE "EXPERIENTIAL QUALITY OF MEANINGFULNESS"

1. For a preliminary discussion of the experience of meaningfulness and its potential role in the justification of the psychoanalytic dream theory see Blass, 1994.

2. The equivalent would be to speak of pain as an experience that, phenomenologically, involves content because it is an experience of there being something painful.

3. As far as I can see, it has been similarly neglected in other relevant fields as well.

4. Of course it is possible that one may connect between ideas in a non-experiential way, but as noted in the previous chapter, this is not the psychoanalytic way. Shortly after Freud's earliest experiments with psychoanalysis it became clear that it is essential to the psychoanalytic process that the connections between the ideas be made in an alive and experiential way. Hence the early importance of transference.

5. Freud had actually attempted to counter the claim that the experience of déjà vu is an illusion. He writes: "It is rather that at such moments something is really touched on which we have already experienced once before, only we cannot consciously remember it because it has never been conscious. To put it briefly, the feeling of '*déjà vu*' corresponds to the recollection of an unconscious phantasy" (Freud, 1901b, p. 266).

Here we see that Freud, in effect, attempts only to counter the argument that déjà vu is an illusion in the sense of it not referring to any real psychic state in the individual. He does not, however, counter the argument that it is an illusion in the sense that it does not refer to anything real in terms of the judgmental statement that it contains regarding the origin of that internal state. On the contrary, by showing the intrapsychic origin of the experience Freud is in fact revealing its illusory nature. Misleading cues lead one to the conclusion that one has been in a certain place previously, although in fact this is not true. The truth is that what had been visited earlier was some unconscious fantasy.

It may also be doubted whether Freud's analysis eliminates the possibility of illusion even in his more limited sense. Demonstrating how in *certain* situations the experience of déjà vu may be tied to unconscious fantasy is an important step, but is clearly not sufficient in itself to counter the more general objection.

6. Of course, one could come up with more bizarre examples of misprocessing of information. For instance, it is possible to imagine that at random time-intervals one comes to false judgments of having been in some place before. This, however, seems to be more far-fetched, and not in line with an attempt to explain an illusion—which is the direction taken in the present argument.

7. Interestingly, Foulkes presents this position in the context of a discussion of why people tend to attribute meaning to the dream.

8. I speak here directly of clinical experience, but one may also include similar evidence that arises from introspection into one's own processes of thought and experience.

9. One may be reminded here of transference relationships. There too there is a current experience of the past. The transference relationship is, however, distinguished from the "experiential quality of meaningfulness" by the fact that the nature of the transference experience per se is not that of "I am now currently experiencing something of the past." Rather, there is a current experience and the individual *understands* that it must be a reliving of a past experience. When the transference experience is indeed an immediate sense of "now I am experiencing something of the past," an experience that goes beyond a conclusion drawn from the contents, then the experience may be considered a specific form of the "experiential quality of meaningfulness." At the end of this chapter I will expand on the issue of variations of the "experiential quality of meaningfulness."

REFERENCES

Altman, L. L. (1969). *The Dream in Psychoanalysis.* New York: Int. Univ. Press.

Anzieu, D. (1986). *Freud's Self-Analysis.* London: Hogarth Press.

Aristotle. (1963). *Nichomachean Ethics.* In *The Philosophy of Aristotle*, ed. R. Bambrough. New York: New American Library.

Arlow, J. A. and Brenner, C. (1964). Dreams and the structural theory. In *Psychoanalytic Concepts and the Structural Theory.* New York: Int. Univ. Press, pp. 114–143.

Atwood, G. E. and Stolorow, R. D. (1984). *Structures of Subjectivity: Explorations in Psychoanalytic Phenomenology.* Hillsdale, N.J.: Analytic Press.

Augustine, St. (1961 [397]). *The Confessions of St. Augustine.* London: Collier Macmillan Publishers.

Balaban, O. (1995). Dream thought. Lecture presented at the 25th Scientific Conference of the Israel Psychological Association, Ben-Gurion University. October, 1995.

Barrat, B. B. (1984). *Psychic Reality and Psychoanalytic Knowing.* Hillsdale, N.J.: Analytic Press.

Basch, M. F. (1976). Theory formation in Chapter VII: A critique. *J. Amer. Psychoanal. Assn.*, 24: 61–100.

Bergmann, M. S. (1966). The intrapsychic and communicative aspects of the dream. *Int. J. Psychoanal.*, 47: 356–363.

Bion,W. R. (1962). *Learning from Experience.* London: Heinemann.

———. (1963). *Elements of Psychoanalysis.* London: Heinemann.

———. (1965). *Transformations.* London: Heinemann.

———. (1970). *Attention and Interpretation.* London: Tavistock.

Blackburn, S. (1984). *Spreading the Word.* Oxford: Oxford Univ. Press.

Blass, R. B. (1993). Die Bedeutung des Traumes: Erschaffen, Entdecken und Erleben. In J. Stork (ed.), Read at "Symbol und Symbolbildung" conference der Poliklinik fur Kinder und Jugendpsychotherapie der Technischen Universtat Munchen. Munich, Germany. September, 1993.

———. (1994). Is psychoanalytic dream interpretation possible? *Pragmatics and Cognition*, 2: 71-94.

———. (2001). The limitations of critical studies of the epistemology of Freud's dream theory and their clinical implications. *Psychoanal. & Contemp. Thought*, 24:115–151.

——— and Blatt, S. J. (1992). Attachment and separateness: A context for the integration of self psychology with object relations theory. *Psychoanal. Study Child*, 47: 189–204.

——— and Simon, B. (1992). Freud on his own mistake(s): The role of seduction in the etiology of neurosis. *Psychiatry and the Humanities*, 12: 160–183.

———. (1994). The value of the historical perspective to contemporary psychoanalysis. *Int. J. Psychoanal.*, 75: 677–694.

Blum, H. P. (1976). The changing uses of dreams in psychoanalytic practice. *Int. J. Psychoanal.*, 57: 315–323.

Bradlow, P. A. (1987). On prediction and the manifest content of the initial dream. In *The Interpretation of Dreams in Clinical Work*, ed. A Rothstein. Madison Conn.: Int. Univ. Press, pp. 155–180.

Brenner, C. (1976). Analysis of dreams, fantasies and similarphenomena. In *Psychoanalytic Technique and Psychic Conflict*. New York: Int. Univ. Press, pp. 133–166.

Breuer, J. and Freud, S. (1895). *Studies on Hysteria. The Standard Edition of the Complete Works of Sigmund Freud, Vol.2*. ed. J. Strchey. London: Hogarth Press.

Carrol, L. (1982 [1872]). *Through the Looking Glass*. In *The Complete Works of Lewis Carrol*. New York: Avenel Books.

Curtis, H. and Sachs, D. (1976). Dialogue on the changing use of dreams in psychoanalytic practice. *Int. J. Psychoanal.*, 57: 343–354.

Dancy, J. (1985). *An Introduction to Contemporary Epistemology*. Oxford: Basil Blackwell.

Danielou, J. (1957). *God and the Ways of Knowing*. New York: Meridian Books.

De Monchaux, C. (1978). Dreaming and the organizing function of the ego. *Int. J. Psychoanal.*, 59: 443–453.

Edelson, M. (1972). Language and dreams: *The Interpretation of Dreams* revisited. *Psychoanal. Study Child*, 27:203–282.

———. (1988). *Psychoanalysis: A Theory in a Crisis*. Chicago: Chicago Univ. Press.

Eliot, G. (1970 [1857]). *Daniel Deronda*. Hammondsworth: Penguin Books.

Erikson, E. H. (1954). The dream specimen of psychoanalysis. *J. Amer. Psychoanal. Assn.*, 2: 5–56.

Ewing, A. C. (1934). *Idealism: A Critical Survey.* London: Methuen.

Eysenck, H. (1985). *The Decline and Fall of the Freudian Empire.* Harmondsworth: Penguin Books.

—— and Wilson, G. C. (1973). *The Experimental Study of Freudian Theories.* London: Methuen.

Fairbairn, W.R.D. (1944). Endopsychic structure considered in terms of object relationships. In *Psychoanalytic Studies of Personality.* London: Tavistock, 1952, pp. 82-136.

Ferenczi, S. (1951). *Theory and Technique in Psychoanalysis.* London: Hogarth Press. pp. 345–350.

Fisher, C. (1978). Experimental and clinical approaches to the mind-body problem through recent research in sleep and dreaming. In *Psychopharmocology and Psychotherapy: Synthesis or Antithesis?*, eds. N. Rosenzweig and H. Griscom. New York: Human Sciences Press, pp. 61–69.

Flanders, S. (1993). Introduction. In *The Dream Discourse Today*, ed. S. Flanders. London: Routledge, 1993, pp. 1–28.

Foulkes, D. (1985). *Dreaming: A Cognitive-Psychological Analysis.* Mahwah, N.J.: Erlbaum.

Freud, S. (1900). *The Interpretation of Dreams.* Vols. 4, 5, ed. J. Strachey, London: Hogarth Press.

——. (1901a). *On Dreams The Standard Edition of The Complete Psychological Works of Sigmund Freud.* Vol. 5, pp. 633–686.

——. (1901b). *The Psychopathology of Everyday Life.* Vol. 6.

——. (1911). *The handling of dream-interpretation in psychoanalysis.* Vol. 12, pp. 89–96.

——. (1914). *On narcissism: An introduction.* Vol. 14, pp. 67–102.

——. (1916a). *Introductory Lectures on Psycho-analysis.* Part I, Lecture IV, parapraxes. Vol. 15, pp. 60–79.

——. (1916b). *Introductory Lectures on Psycho-analysis.* Part II, Lecture VI, the premisses and technique of interpretation. Vol. 15, 100–112.

——. (1923). *Remarks upon the theory and practice of dream-interpretation.* Vol. 19, pp. 109–121.

——. (1933a). *New Introductory Lectures on Psycho-analysis*, Lecture XXIX, revision of the theory of dreams. Vol. 22, pp. 7–30.

——. (1933b). *New Introductory Lectures on Psycho-analysis*, Lecture XXXI, the dissection of the psychical personality. Vol. 22, pp. 57–80.

——. (1933c). *New Introductory Lectures on Psycho-analysis*, Lecture XXXV, the question of a Weltanschauung. Vol. 22, pp. 158–182.

——. (1940). *An Outline of Psychoanalysis.* Vol. 23, pp. 141–207.

——. (1950 [1895]). *A Project for a Scientific Psychology.* Vol. 1, pp. 293–392.

————. (1985). *The Complete Letters of Sigmund Freud to Wilhelm Fliess*, ed. J. M. Masson. Cambridge, Mass: Harvard Univ. Press.

Friedman, L. (1996). Overview: Knowledge and authority in the psychoanalytic relationship. *Psychoanal. Q.*, 65: 254–265.

Gammill, J. (1980). Some reflections on analytic listening and the dream screen. In *The Dream Discourse Today*, ed. S. Flanders. London: Routeledge. 1993, pp. 127–136.

Garma, A. (1966). *The Psychoanalysis of Dreams*. Chicago: Quadrangle Press.

Gay, P. (1988). Freud: *A Life for Our Time*. New York: Norton.

Gill, M. M. (1976). Metapsychology is not psychology. In *Psychology versus Metapsychology: Psychoanalytic Essays in Memory of George S. Klein*, eds. M. M. Gill and P. S. Holzmann. New York: Int Univ. Press, pp. 71–105.

Glucksman, M. L. and Warner, S . L. (eds.) (1987). *Dreams in New Perspective*. New York: Human Sciences Press.

Glymour, C. (1983). The theory of your dreams. In *Physics, Philosophy and Psychoanalysis*, eds. R. Cohen, and L. Laudan. Boston: D. Reidel, pp. 57–71.

Goldberg, A. (1984). The tension between realism and relativism in psychoanalysis. *Psychoanal. Contemp. Thought*, 7:367–386.

Gordon, R. M. (1987) *The Structure of Emotions*. Cambridge: Cambridge Univ. Press.

Green, A. (1967). The analyst, symbolization and absence in the analytic setting. *Int. J. Psychoanal.*, 56: 1–23.

————. (1974). Surface analysis, deep analysis (the role of the preconscious in psychoanalytical technique). *Int. Rev. Psychoanal.*, 1: 415–424.

————. (1977). Conceptions of affect. *Int. J. Psychoanal.*, 58: 129–156.

Greenberg, J. R. and Mitchell, S. A. (1983). *Object Relations in Psychoanalytic Theory*. Cambridge: Harvard Univ. Press.

Greenberg, R. and Pearlman, C. (1975). A psychoanalytic dream continuum; the source and function of dreams. *Int. Rev. Psychoanal.*, 2: 441–448.

————. (1978). If Freud only knew: A reconsideration of psychoanalytic dream theory. *Int. Rev. Psychoanal.*, 5: 71–76.

Greenson, R. R. (1978). The exceptional position of the dream in psychoanalysis. In *Explorations in Psychoanalysis*. New York: Int. Univ. Press.

Grice, H. P. (1975). Logic and conversation. In *Syntax and Semantics, Vol. 3: Speech Acts*, eds. P. Cole and J. L. Morgan. New York: Academic Press, pp. 41–58.

————. (1978). Further notes on logic and conversation. In *Syntax and Semantics, Vol. 9: Pragmatics*, eds. P. Cole and J. L. Morgan. New York: Academic Press, pp. 121–128.

Grinberg, L. (1987). Dreams and acting out. *Psychoanal. Q.*, 56: 155–175.

————. (1990). *The Goals of Psychoanalysis*. London: Karnac Books.

Grinstein, A. (1979). *Sigmund Freud's Dreams*. New York: Int. Univ. Press.

————. (1983). *Freud's Rules of Dream Interpretation.* New York: Int. Univ. Press.

Grotstein, J. S. (1981). Who is the dreamer who dreams the dream and who is the dreamer who understands it? In *Do I Dare Disturb the Universe?*, ed. J. S. Grotstein. Beverly Hills: Caesura Press, pp. 358–416.

————. (1982). Newer perspectives in the object relations theory. *Contemp. Psychoanal.*, 18:43–91.

————. (1983). Some perspectives on self psychology. In *The Future of Psychoanalysis*, ed. A. Goldberg. New York: Int. Univ. Press, pp. 165–201.

————. (1984) A proposed revision of the psychoanalytic concept of primitive mental states. *Contemp. Psychoanal.*, 20:77–119.

Grunbaum, A. (1984). *The Foundation of Psychoanalysis: A Philosophical Critique.* Berkeley: Univ. Calif. Press.

————. (1993). *Validation in the Clinical Theory of Psychoanalysis: A Study in the Philosophy of Psychoanalysis.* Madison: Int. Univ. Press.

Guntrip, H. (1971). *Psychoanalytic Theory, Therapy and the Self.* New York: Basic Books.

Haesler, L. (1994). The role of the dream in present-day psychoanalysis. Lecture presented at the *European Psychoanalytical Federation Scientific Symposium*, Brussels, March 1994.

Hanly. C. (1990). The concept of truth in psychoanalysis. *Int. J. Psychoanal.*, 21: 375–383.

Hartmann, H. (1959). Psychoanalysis as a scientific theory. In *Essays on Ego Psychology*, New York: Int Univ. Press, 1964.

————. (1990). The concept of truth in psychoanalysis. *Int. J. Psychoanal.*, 71: 375–383.

Hobson, A. J. (1988). *The Dreaming Brain.* New York: Basic Books.

————. (1991). Lecture presented at Dartmouth College, Hanover, New Hampshire, McDonnell Neuropsychology Summer School, July 1991.

———— and McCarley, R. W. (1977). The brain as a dream state generator: An activation synthesis hypothesis of the dream process. *Amer. J. Psychiatry*, 134: 1335–1348.

Hoffmann, I. Z. (1991). Discussion: Toward a social-constructivist view of the psychoanalytic situation. *Psychoanal. Dialogues*, 1: 74–105.

Home, H. J. (1966). The concept of mind. *Int. J. Psychoanal.*, 47: 42–49.

Hook, S. (ed) (1959). *Psychoanalysis, Scientific Method and Philosophy*, New York: New York Univ. Press.

Jones, E. (1953). *The Life and Work of Sigmund Freud*, vol. 1. New York: Basic Books.

Kanzer, M. (1955). The communicative function of the dream. *Int. J. Psychoanal.*, 36: 260–266.

Kaplan, D. M. (1989). The place of the dream in psychotherapy. *Bull. Menninger Clinic*, 58: 1–17.

Khan, M. M. R. (1962). Dream psychology and the evaluation of the psychoanalytic situation. In *The Privacy of the Self.* New York: Int. Univ. Press, 1974, pp. 27–41.

———. (1972). The use and abuse of the dream in psychic experience. In *The Privacy of the Self.* New York : Int. Univ. Press, 1974, pp. 306–315.

———. (1974). *The Privacy of the Self.* New York: Int. Univ. Press.

———. (1976). The changing use of dreams in psychoanalysis. *Int. J. Psychoanal.*, 57: 325–330.

———. (1979). *Alienation in Perversions.* New York: Int. Univ. Press.

———. (1983a). Beyond the dreaming experience. In *Hidden Selves.* New York: Int. Univ. Press, pp. 254–271.

———. (1983b). *Hidden Selves.* New York: Int. Univ. Press.

Klauber, J. (1967). Reporting dreams in psychoanalysis. In *Difficulties in the Analytic Encounter.* New York: Jason Aronson, 1981, pp. 3–24.

———. (1981). Introduction. In *Difficulties in the Analytic Encounter.* New York: Jason Aronson, pp. xiii–xxxii.

Klein, G. S. (1976). *Psychoanalytic Theory: An Exploration of Essentials.* New York: Int. Univ. Press.

Kohut, H. (1971). *The Analysis of the Self.* New York: Int. Univ. Press.

———. (1977). *The Restoration of the Self.* New York: Int. Univ. Press.

———. (1983). Selected problems of self psychological theory. In *Reflections on Self Psychology*, ed. J. D. Lichtenberg and S. Kaplan. Hillsdale, N.J.: Analytic Press, pp. 387–416.

Kris, A. (1982). *Free Associations.* New Haven: Yale Univ. Press.

Kris, E. (1954). New contributions to the study of Freud's "The Interpretation of Dreams"; A critical essay. *J. Amer. Psychoanal. Assn.*, 2:180–191.

Kubie, L. (1966). A reconsideration of thinking, the dream process, and "the dream." *Psychoanl. Q.*, 35: 191–198.

Kulka, R. (1994). The psychoanalyst's mind from listening to interpretation: Will psychoanalysis evolve from individuality to subjectivity? In *The Analyst's Mind from Listening to Interpretation*, ed. IPAC Amsterdam. London: The IPA Press.

Labruzza, A. L. (1978). The activation-synthesis hypothesis of dreams: A theoretical note. *Amer. J. Psychiatry.* 135: 1536–1538.

Lehrer, K. (1974). *Knowledge.* Oxford: Clarendon Press.

Lewin, B. D. (1946). Sleep, the mouth, and the dream screen. *Psychoanalytic Q.*, 15: 419–434.

———. (1953). Reconsideration of the dream screen. *Psychoanal. Q.*, 22: 174–199.

———. (1958). *Dreams and the Uses of Regression.* New York: Int. Univ. Press.

Masson, J. M. (1984). *The Assault on Truth*. New York: Farrar, Straus & Giroux.

McCarley, R. W. and Hobson, J. A. (1977). The neurobiological origins of psychoanalytic dream theory. *Amer. J. Psychiatry*, 134: 1211–1221.

McLeod, M. N. (1992). The evolution of Freud's theory about dreaming. *Psychoanal. Q.*, 61: 37–64.

Meltzer, D. (1981). The Kleinian expansion of Freud's metapsychology. *Int. J. Psychoanal.*, 62: 177–185.

———. (1984). *Dream-Life: A Reexamination of the Psychoanalytical Theory and Technique*. Perthshire: Clunie Press.

Moore, M. (1983). The nature of psychoanalytic explanation. In *Mind and Medicine: Expalantion and Evaluation in Psychiatry and the Biomedical Sciences*, ed. L. Laudan. Berkley: Univ. California Press, pp 5–78.

Nagel, E. (1959). Methodological issues in psychoanalytic theory. In *Psychoanalysis, Scientific Method and Philosophy.*, ed. S. Hook. New York: Grove Press, 1960, pp, 38–56.

Nagera, H., Baker, S., Colonna, A., Edgecumbe, R., Holder, A, Kearney, L., Kawenoka, M., Legg, C., Meers, D., Neurath, L., and Rees, K., (1969). *Basic Psychoanalytic Concepts on the Theory of Dreams*. New York: Basic Books.

Ornstein, P. H. (1987). On self-state dreams in the psychoanalytic treatment process. In *The Interpretation of Dreams in Clinical Work*, ed. A. Rothstein. Madison Conn.: Int. Univ. Press, pp. 87–104.

Palombo, S. (1978). *Dreaming and Memory*. New York: Basic Books.

Pessoa, F. (1991). *The Book of Disquiet*. New York: Pantheon Books.

Peterfreund, E. (1971). *Information, Systems, and Psychoanalysis*. New York: Int. Univ. Press.

Plata-Mujica, C. (1976). Discussion of 'The changing use of dreams in psychoanalysis.' *Int. J. Psychoanal.*, 57: 335–341.

Pontalis, J. -B. (1973). Dream-makers. In *Frontiers in Psychoanalysis*. New York: Int. Univ. Press.

———. (1974a). Dream as an object *Int. Rev. Psychoanal.*, 1: 125–133.

———. (1974b). The dream: Between Freud and Breton. In *Frontiers in Psychoanalysis*. New York: Int. Univ. Press, 1981, pp. 49–55.

———. (1981). Between the dream as object and the dream as text. In *Frontiers in Psychoanalysis*. New York: Int. Univ. Press., pp. 23–55.

Popper, K. R. (1963). *Conjectures and Refutations: the Growth of Scientific Knowledge*. New York: Basic Books.

Pulver, S. E. (1987). The manifest dream in psychoanalysis. *J. Amer. Psychoanal. Assn.*, 35: 99–118.

Quine, W. V. O. (1960). *Word and Object*. Cambridge: MIT Press.

Rangell, L. (1987). Historical perspectives and current status of the interpretation of dreams in clinical work. In *The Interpretation of Dreams in Clinical Work*, ed. A. Rothstein. Madison Conn.: Int. Univ. Press, pp. 3–24.

Renik, O, (1993). Analytic interaction: Conceptualizing technique in light of the analyst's irreducible subjectivity. *Psychoanal. Q.*, 62: 553–571.

———. (1998). The analyst's subjectivity and the analyst's objectivity. *Int. J. Psychoanal.*, 79: 487–497.

Rescher, N. (1973). *The Coherence Theory of Truth*. Oxford: Clarendon Press.

Ricouer, P. (1970). *Freud, and Philosophy*, London: Yale University Press.

———. (1974). *The Conflict of Interpretations*. Evanston, Ill.: Northwestern Univ. Press.

———. (1981). *Hermeneutics and the Human Sciences*. New York: Cambridge Univ. Press.

Rothstein, A. (1987). Conclusion. In *The Interpretation of Dreams in Clinical Work.*, ed. A. Rothstein. Madison: Int. Univ. Press, pp. 197–204.

Rycroft, C. (1966). Causes and meanings. In *Psychoanalysis Observed*, ed. C. Rycroft. London: Constable, pp. 7–22.

———. (1979). *The Innocence of Dreams*. London: Hogarth Press.

Schachter, S. and Singer, J. E. (1962). Cognitive, social and physiological determinants of emotional state. *Psychological Review*, 69: 379–399.

Schafer, R. (1976). *A New Language for Psychoanalysis*. New Haven: Yale Univ. Press.

———. (1978). *Language and Insight*. New Have: Yale Univ. Press.

———. (1983). *The Analytic Attitude*. New York: Basic Books.

Schlick, M. (1959). Positivism and realism. In *Logical Positivism*, ed. A. J. Ayer. New York: Macmillan Co., pp. 86–87.

Schur, M. (1972). *Freud: Living and Dying*. London: Hogarth Press.

Segal, H. (1986). The function of dreams. *The Work of Hanna Segal*. London: Free Association, pp. 89–97.

Shanon, B. (1990). Why are dreams cinematographic? *Metaphor and Symbolic Activity*, 5: 235–248.

———. Eifermann, R. (1984). Dreamreporting discourse. *Text* 4: 369–379.

Sherwood, M. (1969). *The Logic of Explanation in Psychoanalysis*. New York: Academic Press.

Shope, R. K. (1973). Freud's concepts of meaning. *Psychoanal. Contemp. Science.*, 2: 276–302.

Sloane, P. (1979). *Psychoanalytic Understanding of the Dream*. New York: Jason Aronson.

Spence, D. P. (1981). Toward a theory of dream interpretation. *Psychoanal. Contemp. Thought.* 4: 383–405.

———. (1982a). *Narrative Truth and Historical Truth*. New York: Norton.

————. (1982b). Narrative truth and theoretical truth. *Psychoanal. Q.*, 51: 43–69.

Steele, R. S. (1979). Psychoanalysis and hermeneutics. *Int. Rev. Psychoanal.*, 6: 389–412.

Stolorow, R. D. and Atwood, G. E. (1982). Psychoanalytic phenomenology of the dream. *Annual of Psychoanalysis*, 10: 208–220.

Strenger, C. (1991). *Between Hermeneutics and Science: An Essay on the Epistemology of Psychoanalysis*. Madison, Wis.: Int. Univ. Press.

Tillich, P. (1957). *Dynamics of Faith*. New York: Harper & Row.

Tolpin, P. (1983). Self psychology and the interpretation of dreams. In *The Future of Psychoanalysis*, ed. A. Goldberg. New York: Int.Univ. Press, pp. 254–271.

Vogel, G. W. (1978). An alternative view of the neurobiology of dreaming. *Amer. J. Psychiatry*, 135: 1531–1535.

Waelder, R. (1960). *Basic Theory of Psychoanalysis*. New York: Int. Univ. Press.

Waldhorn, H. F. (1967). *Reporter: Indications for Psychoanalysis: The Place of Dreams in Clinical Psychoanalysis*. Monograph II of the Kris Study group of the New York Psychoanalytic Institute. New York: Int. Univ. Press.

Wallerstein, R. S. (1964). The role of prediction in theory building in psychoanalyis. *J. Amer. Psychonal. Assn.*, 12: 675–691.

————. (1976). Psychoanalysis as a science. In *Psychology versus Metapsychology: Psychoanalytic Essays in Memory of George S. Klein.*, eds. M. M. Gill and P. S. Holzmann. New York: Int. Univ. Press, pp. 198–228.

————. (1986). Psychoanalysis as a science: A respone to the new challenges. *Psychoanal. Q.*, 55: 414–451.

Welsh, A. (1994). *Freud's Wishful Dream Book*. Princeton: Princeton Univ. Press.

Winnicott, D. W. (1958). *Collected Papers: Through Paediatrics to Psychoanalysis*. London: Tavistock.

————. (1971). Dreaming, fantasying and living. In *Playing and Reality*. London: Tavistock. pp. 26–37.

Index

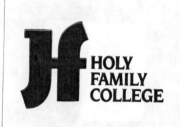

**HOLY
FAMILY
COLLEGE**